STANDING POSTURES

JEREMY CORNISH, LAC.

Mountain Shadow Publishing
513 w. 87th st
Naperville, IL 60565

All photos and images by Marissa Cornish, except headshot by Stephen Carrera.

Please note: The creators and publishers of this book disclaim any liability for loss in connection with following any of the practices, exercises, and advice contained herein. To reduce the chance of injury or any other harm, the reader should consult a professional before undertaking this or any other martial arts, movement, meditative arts, health, or exercise program. The instructions and advice printed in this book are not in any way intended as a substitute for medical, mental, or emotional counseling with a licensed physician or healthcare provider.

To my family of teachers.

Contents

Disclaimer

For those with any major health concerns, it is recommended that you talk with your doctor before beginning any exercise routine.

This practice should generally not be painful.

This practice is about personal empowerment. Listen to your body, and trust your intuition. If something doesn't feel quite right it probably isn't. Injuring yourself is counterproductive, especially for a longevity exercise.

You are responsible for your own safety during practice.

The Nature of This Book

This book is a training manual, a pragmatic guide to implementing practices and concepts from Eastern Medicine and Martial Arts to enhance your experience of life. I've had great teachers, and been exposed to a lot of "pearls of wisdom." I've done my best here to discern the thread that unites those pearls, and present it here for you.

This is not a scholarly text. You will not find footnotes or a bibliography. There are already plenty of texts that approach these arts from a more academic, historical, or research-based angle. Most of the material in this book comes from oral transmission and my own and my students' experience. I have not included much of my own biography or stories of my teachers' special abilities. I'm assuming you're less interested in how these exercises changed my life, more how they can change yours.

I realized years ago that there is no "one right way" to practice. Much like medicine, the correctness of the method depends entirely on how well it helps you achieve your specific goals.

Teachers are a vital link in the chain of collective wisdom. The best ones help to lay an adaptable foundation upon which true skill can be built. To sincerely progress, there comes a point when your body becomes your true teacher, and you are your own master.

The lineage of the transmission is nowhere near as important as the information itself. The attitude of the practitioner matters even more.

Benefits of Standing Postures

Standing Postures are some of the simplest, most effective ways to strengthen the body and mind. These types of exercises are one of my go-to "homework assignments" for patients in between acupuncture sessions.

The benefits can be profound. Depending on which posture you are practicing, there will be differing amounts of physical stress on the body. Regardless of the amount of physical stress, the goal of practice is to seek relaxation and acceptance of the position, training your nervous system to change a potentially stressful experience into a welcome, relaxing one. This is a valuable skill with vast implications.

Physically, these postures tend to develop suppleness, increase circulation, and strengthen the joints. By maintaining a posture, we allow our soft tissue to relax and align. It is hard to maintain poor alignment for long. The soreness and muscular fatigue you'll feel are actually messages from your body teaching you how to properly hold yourself. Listen.

Mentally, when we practice, we are exercising certain skills such as willpower, discipline, and focus. Approaching practice with a curious, interested, nonjudgmental state of mind is advised. We get good at what we practice. Practice often creates an internal environment more conducive to creativity, inspiration, and performance enhancement. Many high level artists, athletes, and business professionals have benefited from the auxiliary benefits that come with consistent practice.

You may also notice your personality changes a bit. Generally, those who meditate regularly have less turbulent emotional ups and downs, and are more able to stay centered through the twists and turns of life. Most practitioners tend to be bothered less and less by personal dramas. External events tend to have less emotional impact as the internal center becomes stronger.

Also, I have found Standing to be especially helpful for recuperating from jet-lag. Skip the coffee and melatonin. Next time you travel, try 10-15 minutes of Standing on Stake (page 80) once you reach your destination.

Modular Thinking

There is an ongoing tug of war between structure and freedom. Too many rules and guidelines will leave little opportunity for spontaneity and creativity. Yet without structure we are lost. There would be no discipline, and no way to gauge progress, or to know if our practice is taking us where we want to go.

A resilient system allows for the balance of these two forces. Modular Thinking is the ability to identify the broad stroke categorical elements of the structure, and then flesh those bones out with specifics that get the job done. If you've ever made a sandwich, then you already know how to do this.

Let's identify the categorical elements that compose a sandwich.

- Bread
- Meat
- Cheese
- Condiments
- Extras

Another way to put this is:

Sandwich = Bread + Meat + Cheese + Condiments + Extras

Each of these required elements could be satisfied by a variety of actual substances.

Your bread could be sourdough, whole grain, bun, focaccia, etc. Meat could be ham, roast beef, turkey, chicken breast, or completely omitted in the case of vegetarians. The cheese could be cheddar, swiss, brie, etc. Condiments could be mustard, mayo, thousand island etc. Extras is the fun category that allows for special additions such as tomatoes, onions, banana peppers, a fried egg, pickles, etc.

In this way, a simple concept (the sandwich) is made up of a few key categorical elements. Those categories each contain a variety of substances to choose from. The permutations are endless. Variations on a theme. Modular thinking allows you to eat a sandwich every day, without ever eating the same one twice.

Of course not every combination is necessarily delicious. Though there are a few famous combos that have earned their own name. The Club. The Reuben. BLT.

And there is also the famous Grilled Cheese, which only pulls from two (three if you add tomatoes) of the required categories, but still qualifies as a sandwich. That in itself tells us something about the weight of the categories in terms of importance.

Bread is what makes a sandwich. Without bread the meat, cheese, condiments and extras just sit in a pile on a plate. The key defining element is gone. With a little nudging, this heap could become something else. A salad. Or a deli tray. But not a sandwich, not without bread.

With some substitution, using a pita, tortilla, or big piece of lettuce instead of the bread, we no longer have a sandwich, we have a wrap. Something similar, but no longer a sandwich.

Modular Thinking is extremely empowering because it allows us to improvise and adapt to changing circumstances while staying true to our underlying structure and vision.

This book is designed to encourage Modular Thinking around your practice. When you design your standing practice, consider the following categorical elements:

- Warming Up
- Stretching
- Posture
- Extras
- Closing

Practice = Warmups + Stretches + Posture + Extras + Close

Warming Up can include the Counterswing, the Lift and Drop, or Bouncing. There is a list of stretches in the Dao Yin section. Posture is further composed of a combination of elements (Upper Body Postures + Stances) that you can mix and match. Extras include the Qi Gong, Nei Gong, and Shen Gong described throughout. My favorite Closing is Scooping the Moon (page 40) followed by standing quietly for a moment.

Feel free to add any other exercises to these categories as you build your practice. By rotating out specific exercises within any category, you can create a dynamic practice that never gets boring, while continuing to progress on your path.

Just as bread is the most important categorical element of a sandwich, the standing posture is the most important part of your standing practice. If you're short on time, skip the warmups. Keep the posture.

Basics

Clothes should be loose and comfortable. There is no need to buy a special shiny silk suit for this, unless that's already your kind of thing. Tight belts and uncomfortable shoes are something to generally be avoided in life, even more so for this.

Some people really like to practice barefoot. Others prefer shoes. Both can be good depending on the environment. If you're outside in cold damp grass, it might be better to wear shoes than to have wet numb feet at the end of practice.

That being said, there may be some value to standing outside for 10 minutes every morning in your underwear to tune your immune system to the weather of the season. By the way, don't try that if you're sick, or have immune issues. See an acupuncturist or herbalist first to get yourself back to basic health.

Breathing is done primarily through the nose. Let each inhalation softly expand the lower abdomen, and each exhalation slightly draw the abdomen back in.

Eyes open or closed. It's up to you. If open, let your gaze be soft.

Structured Practice

Typically, it's best to move around a bit before standing still. Just a few minutes of the Counterswing (page 20) and/or Bouncing (page 22) beforehand can make the Standing so much easier.

When you are holding your posture, set a timer. That way you don't have to busy yourself counting breaths, or become distracted by having to check a clock. The alarm will go off when it's time. Patience is part of this practice. There is nowhere else to be, and nothing else to be doing. Deconstructing the layer of the mind that is constantly worried about time is incredibly difficult, but incredibly rewarding.

Hold the postures for as long as you like. 2 minutes is a good start. Each time you practice add another minute, until you're in the sweet spot. For the deeper, more physically challenging postures like Horse Stance (page 82), 5 minutes is a solid practice.

More neutral positions like Standing on Stake (page 80) lend themselves well to longer times. For these types of postures, 20-30 minutes is an admirable and very achievable goal. If you'd like to go longer, be my guest.

Many people enjoy practicing Standing on Stake for an hour or more.

Usually once you've passed the 15 minute mark, you feel such a sense of mental clarity that when the timer goes off you'll actually feel a twinge of disappointment. It's over too soon. Be aware of that reaction. Set it for longer next time.

When the timer does go off, don't lose your focus. Calmly and slowly float the hands up over the head and conclude your practice with at least three repetitions of Scooping the Moon (page 40), remembering to let your body draw the energy from the center of the Earth, guiding it through your entire being, and out into the space around you.

Warming Up

Standing still can be challenging at first. The mind and body are accustomed to constant motion. Get the twitches, fidgets, and restless urges out of the way beforehand and your Standing practice will be much more enjoyable.

Throughout the warm-ups, remember to breathe smoothly and deeply from the belly, and keep the body as relaxed and soft as possible.

The Counterswing

Begin this exercise by standing naturally, with the feet approximately shoulder width apart. Make sure you have room around yourself so that you won't hit anyone or anything. As you float your arms up and out to the sides, your body makes a "T" shape. Now let the arms fall freely downwards, turning your body to one side so that they naturally swing back up into a twisted "T." Reverse the motion to get back to your original "T" shape, and then repeat for the other side.

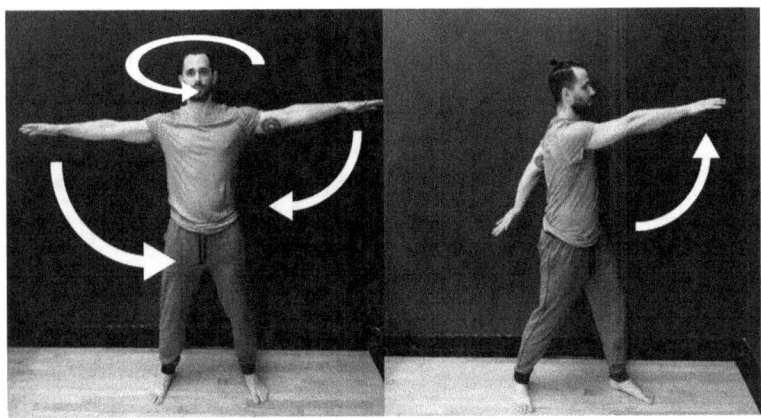

Once you understand the basic mechanics of the arms and the core, this exercise should become almost effortless, as you develop a rhythm like a pendulum. The raising and lowering of the arms is driven by the twisting of the body, letting gravity do the work.

As this becomes a more comfortable movement, you'll notice that your legs and feet naturally pivot during the twisting. Remember to keep the knees soft (slightly bent), integrate the entire body into this relaxed movement, breathe smoothly, and keep swinging for 1 to 5 minutes. Then move into the Lift and Drop.

Lift and Drop

Begin in a neutral stance. As you slowly inhale, become as tall and expanded as possible. Let the spine extend, the chest open, look upwards, and press up onto your tiptoes. The inhalation is a stretch for the front of the body, and everything expands during this phase.

As you exhale, allow the body to become loose like a rag doll, and drop into a relaxed, soft stance. It may take some practice to get the feel for this.

The Lift and Drop works by propagating a wave up the spine. This waving motion helps to warm and increase the blood circulation around the spine. Moving like this also helps the circulation of the cerebrospinal fluid.

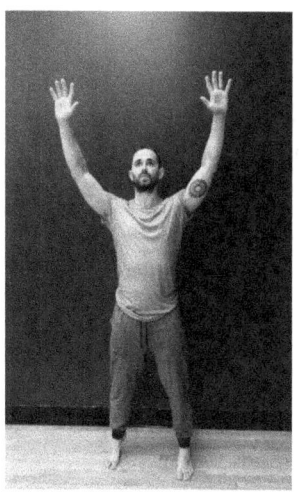 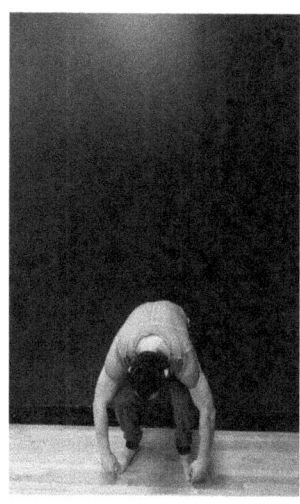

Perform the Lift and Drop 3 times, and then transition directly into the next warm-up, Bouncing.

Bouncing

Keeping your feet on the ground, allow the entire body to oscillate up and down in a gentle bouncing movement. Make sure not to abuse the knees during this exercise. As with the Counterswing, Bouncing should feel very natural, with the body relaxed, and gravity doing the work. As you bounce, notice areas of the body that are restricted. Let the shoulders move. For women, the breasts should be moving, and for men the testes. This may seem embarrassing at first, but there's nothing inherently sexual about this exercise. Stagnation is not conducive to good health. It is especially important to create movement in

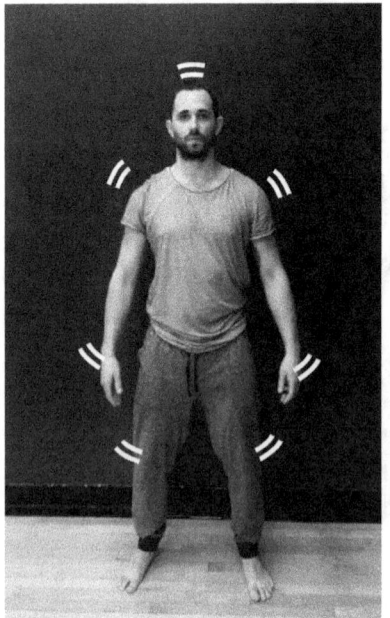

areas of the body that normally stay still or confined.

Keep the breathing smooth and easy. Continue gently bouncing for 2 to 5 minutes.

Bouncing helps to release muscular tension, and also gently compresses the bones of the skeleton, creating stronger, denser bones. Bouncing also helps fluids to circulate.

Dao Yin

After you've done some warm-ups, the muscles will respond better to stretching. Dao Yin means not only stretching, but stretching and guiding. One of the key takeaways from this is to stay expanded as you stretch. Don't crunch yourself.

Neck

Standing comfortably slowly let the right ear drop towards the right shoulder, allowing the left side of the neck to open up. Make sure to keep your shoulders low and relaxed, especially the left one. If you'd like to enhance this stretch, you can always grab your left wrist with your right hand behind your back, pulling the arms and shoulders down. Hold this stretch for a few breaths, consciously letting the energy move into and through the stretch.

Then, slowly let the chin roll down towards the chest. Really take your time with this transition, allowing the stretch to migrate from the side to the back of the neck, as you eventually let your head hang down in front. Take a few breaths here, letting the spine relax and become full of energy. Then slowly float the head back up to the center. Repeat on the other side.

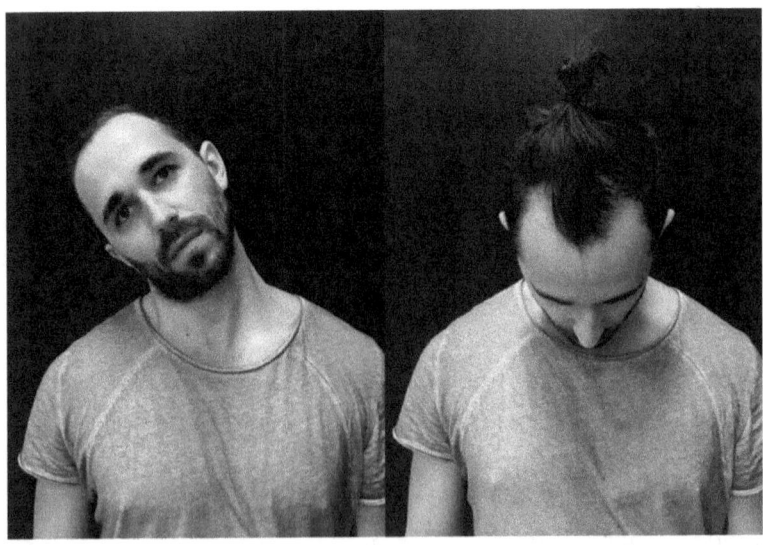

Flanks

Once you've finished both sides of the neck and floated your head back to the center, float your arms up over your head, linking your hands. Bring your feet close together. As you inhale, get very tall and reach up towards the sky. As you exhale, push your right hip out to the right as you extend your arms out to the left. This creates an excellent stretch along the ride side of the torso (the flank). Try to keep the arms extended so as not to kink your left side. Hold this position for a few breaths, then use your core to straighten up. Repeat on the other side.

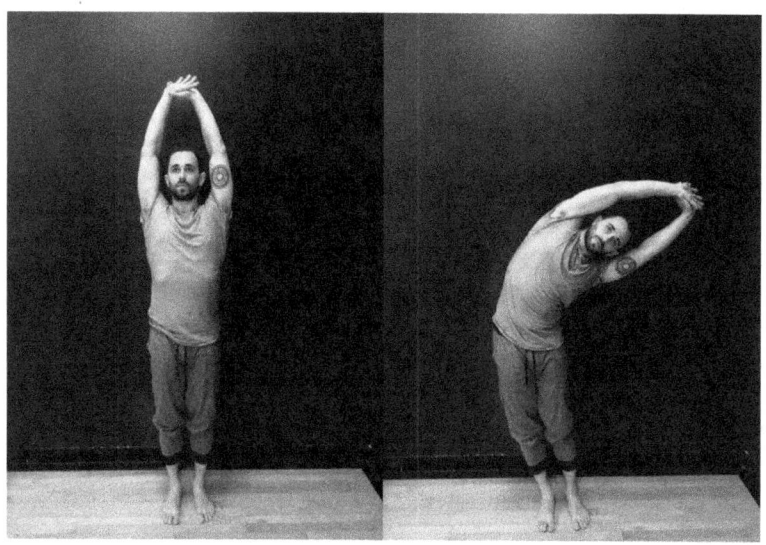

Rhomboids and Lats

The rhomboid muscles are a common place of tension, often leading to neck and upper back pain. These muscles are on the upper back, and they run horizontally between the scapulae and the spine. They are nestled underneath the trapezius. The best way to release these muscles is direct acupuncture. Skilled massage therapists can get them as well. The upper back in general is a difficult area to stretch, though there are ways. Learning this stretch requires that you feel inside your body and really use your awareness as well as the Dao Yin concept of guiding energy. You may have to play with the angles to find the position that engages your back the right way.

Make sure your feet are shoulder width, and bring your hands out in front of you at chest height, palms pointed out. Grab the right wrist with your left hand, and reach your arms forward while rounding out your upper back. This should take the slack out of the shoulder blades, and create a stretch in the rhomboid area.

Maintaining the roundness in the upper back, and without losing the stretch, slowly tilt your right arm so that the fingers point to the ground, and the elbow points to the sky. You might raise your right shoulder as well, allowing the stretch to expand into that area.

Keeping the stretch, turn from your waist towards the left. You might feel the stretch now spreading down the lower trapezius and latisissimus towards the right hip.

Lastly, allow your body to fold, so that the hands trace the area over the outside of the left leg. This creates a massive stretch that encompasses the right side of the back from rhomboids to hips. Hold this position for a few breaths, and then gradually let the upper body transition into a forward fold. Take a few breaths here, then bend your knees, and slowly stand up with your legs. Repeat on the other side.

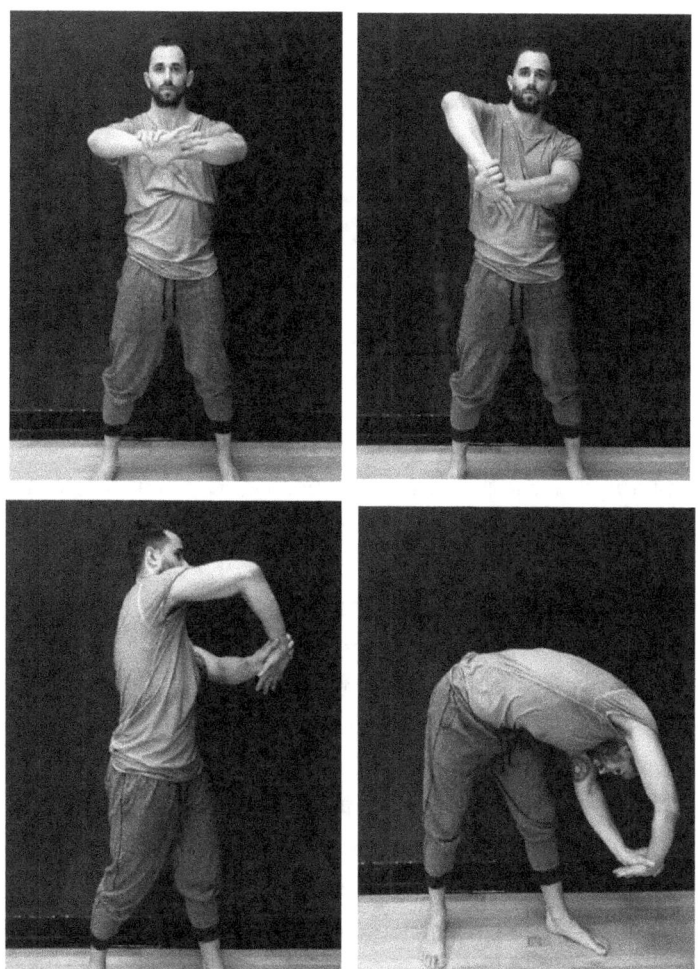

Rotator Cuff

The rotator cuff is another area that is prone to injury and difficult to stretch without internal awareness.

Starting from standing, step the feet apart so they are double shoulder width. Let the knees bend, sinking into a deep, wide squat. If your knees give you pain, don't go as deeply until the strength is built back up. Place the palms on the insides of the thighs, close to the knees. Keeping your right elbow relatively straight, allow your right hand to pivot on your thigh, fingers pointing towards your body, as you drop your right shoulder in front of you. The straighter (not locked) that you keep the right elbow, the more you'll get the stretch. You know you have this one when you feel as if your right shoulder is being twisted and wrung out.

Hold for a few breaths, then come back to the center and repeat on the other side.

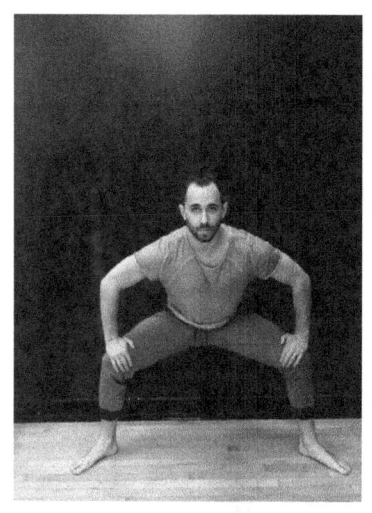

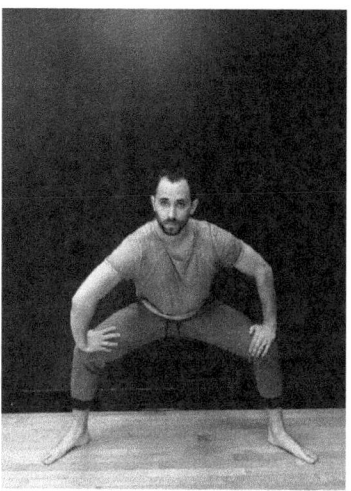

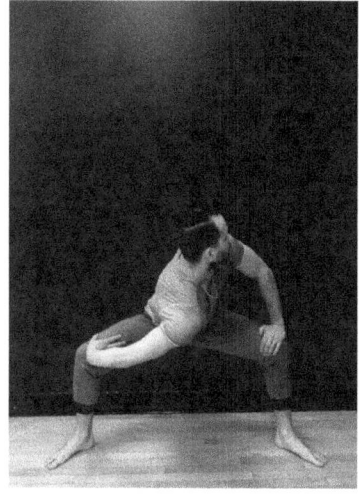

I.T. Band & Hamstrings

The Iliotibial (I.T.) Band is a taught strap of connective tissue that runs down the outside of your thigh. This is another of those body areas that so often gets overlooked in stretching.

Bring all of your weight to the right foot. Lightly place the left heel on the ground about shoulder width from your right foot. Turn your left toes out towards your back. This creates a rotation in the left leg that opens the hips. Keeping the left leg extended, though not locked, sink into your right leg, allowing the outside of the left leg to stretch and open. If you feel it on the back of the leg rather than the side, you are stretching your hamstrings, which is also a good thing to stretch. To focus the stretch on the side, make sure the left foot stays rotated out. You may have to play with the angle of rotation, as well as the angle of how you sit back into the stretch.

Hold the stretch for a few breaths, and repeat on the other side.

Another great way to soften the I.T. Band is to go after it with a foam roller.

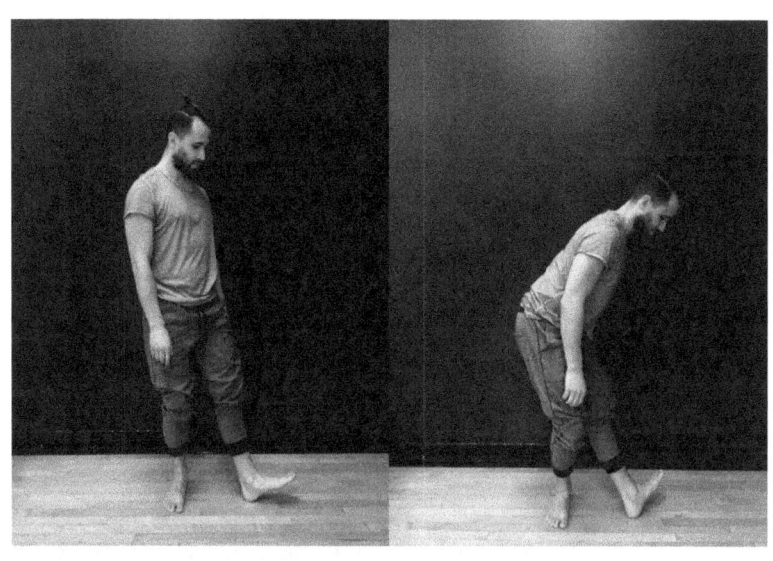

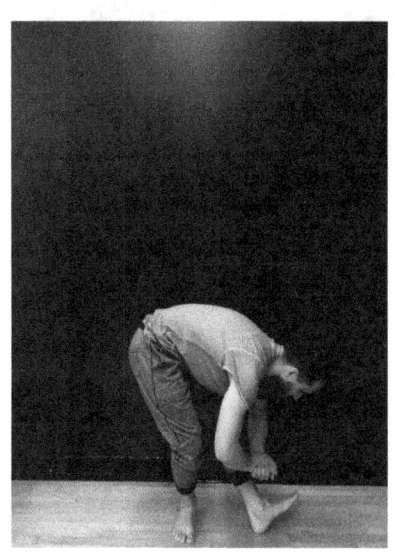

Forward Fold

From a neutral stance, inhale as you let the arms float above the head, extending your spine so that you become as tall as possible. As you exhale, keep your spine long and fold out from the waist until the upper body hangs relaxed like a rag doll. Consciously soften and relax your spine, letting the weight of your head provide natural traction. Imagine all of the tension in your spine dripping downwards and out the top of your head into the ground. Hold this stretch for a few breaths, then bend your knees, look up, and stand up with your legs.

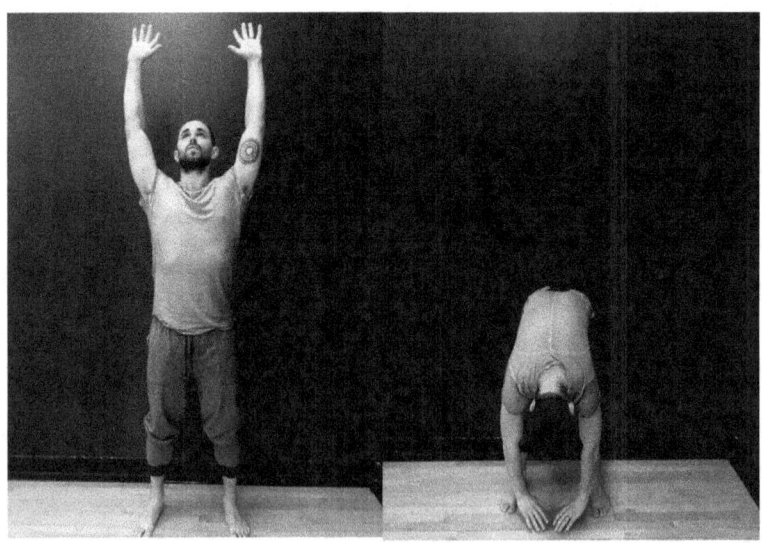

Qi Gong

Qi Gong

Qi Gong ("Energy Cultivation") exercises teach us to be aware of the energy inside of and around our bodies. There are thousands of styles of Qi Gong, each with their own quirks and merits. For the purposes of this book, though, we only need to examine two very common Qi Gong exercises, the Qi Ball and the Qi Bubble.

The Qi Ball
Bring the hands in front of your body as if you are holding an invisible ball. The hands face each other so that the centers of the palms are pointed at each other. Imagine a sphere of energy between your hands, and the axis of that sphere is the tube that connects your two palms.

As you inhale, allow the hands to move slightly apart, expanding the ball. Feel the tug in the space between your palms. As you exhale, press the palms slightly closer to each other, compressing the ball. Feel the pressure in the space between your palms as you squeeze the axis of the sphere.

Make sure you follow a cycle of expansion and *compression*, which builds a charge.

Thinking in terms of expansion and *contraction* will dissipate the energy before it can build up.

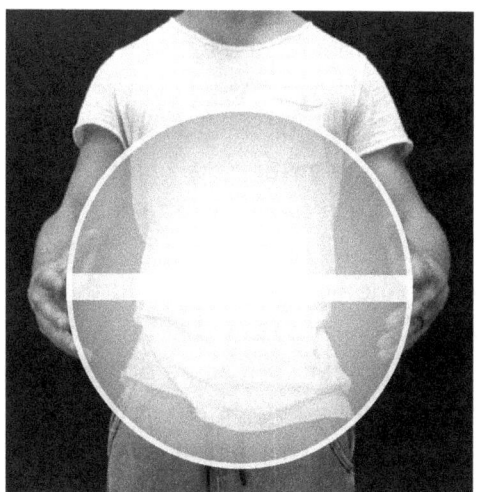

The Qi Ball with an axis connecting the centers of the palms.

The Qi Bubble

Once you have the hang of the Qi Ball, you can move on to the Qi Bubble. The Bubble is basically a Qi Ball so big that it envelops your whole body.

One way to get the feel for the Qi Bubble is to start with a Qi Ball between the hands. As you inhale, let the ball expand about 6-8 inches on each side as the hands move apart. When you exhale, keep the hands in their new position, and simply press against the surface of the ball.

Inhale again, expanding the ball even further, then hold and press during the exhalation. In this way the ball is being inflated with every breath. At some point the ball will be so big that your arms are outstretched at the end of their range of motion. When this happens, inhale once more, and as you exhale, turn the palms to face away from the body. Imagine that you are now inside of a Qi Bubble that envelops your whole body. Feel the surface of the bubble against your palms.

See the following four photos.

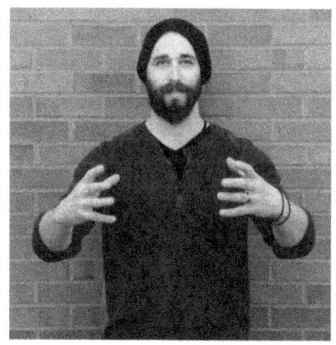
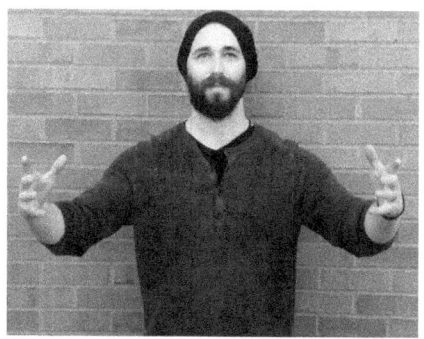
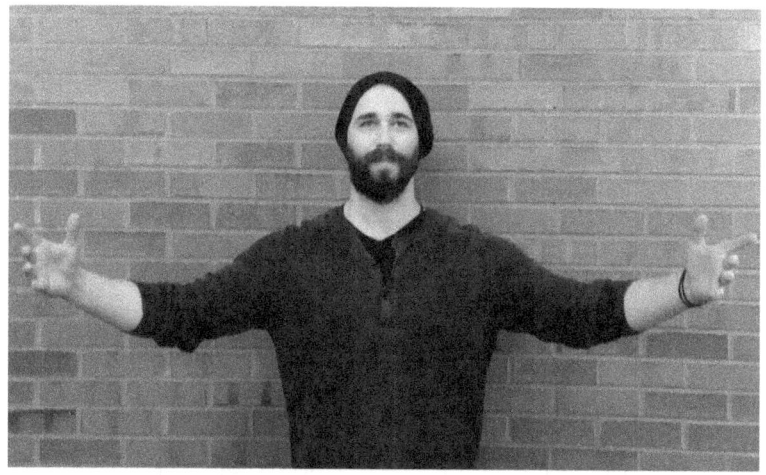
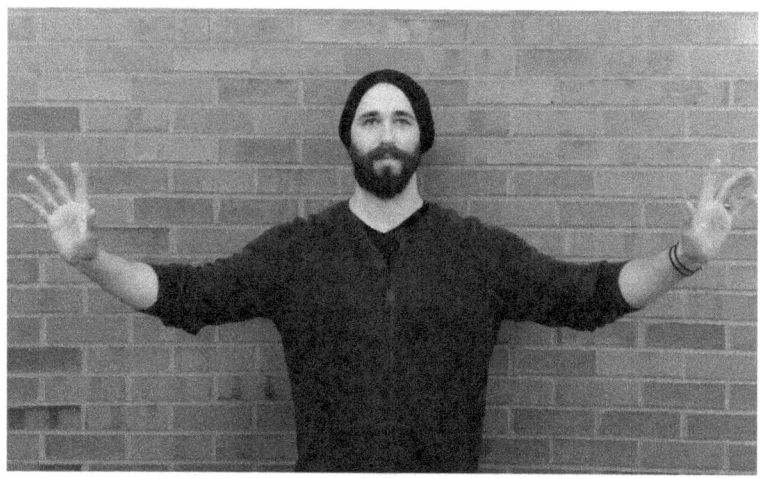

Scooping the Moon

This exercise combines the Qi Ball with the Qi Bubble, and is highly effective for establishing your space and closing up a practice session.

From a neutral stance, make a Qi Ball in front of your lower abdomen. Inhale slowly as you lift the ball up the center of your body, all the way over your head, but not so high that tension is created in the shoulders. As you do this, imagine the energy ball is bringing pure energy from the center of the Earth up through your entire body. Let your face and eyes float a bit to follow the hands.

As you exhale, slowly turn the palms to face forward as you gently glide the arms out to the sides and down, imagining all that energy distributing itself throughout your entire body, and also charging the field around you. Let your head and gaze return to a neutral position.

Repeat for a total of 3-9 times, and then stand comfortably. Close your eyes, take a few more breaths, and notice how your body feels. You may also get a sense of the space around your body.

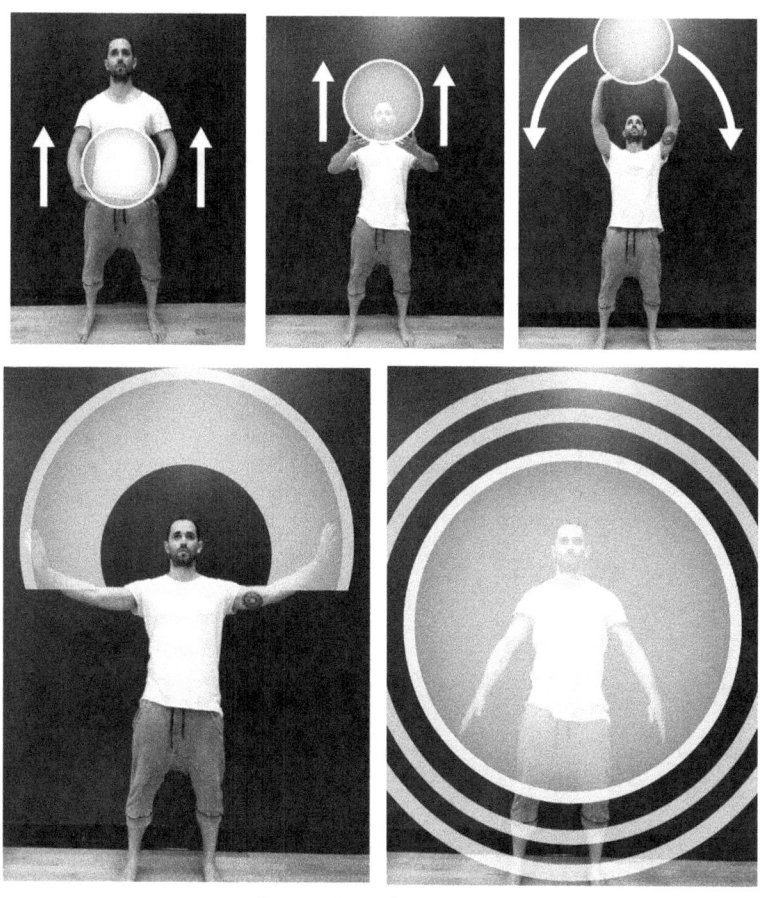

Scooping the Moon.

Postures and Stances

Standing Postures

There are a wide variety of Standing Postures that have roots in all manner of Yogic, Martial and Meditative traditions. In this chapter we will look at a few of these classical favorites.

We'll spend some time in this chapter exploring various upper body and lower body positions. These are the elements of the Standing Postures. You can create your own by simply mixing and matching.

The postures presented here are merely suggestions. I find it's best to let the posture emerge naturally from a moving practice. For example, if you practice Scooping the Moon (page 40) extremely slowly, you'll find certain points within that motion that make excellent holding positions.

If you have a movement vocabulary from another practice such as Tai Chi or dance, you may choose to hold your body in the pinnacle position of one of those techniques. The posture emerges from the motion.

The temptation to collect postures and techniques can be strong, but I will say here that I believe the value of practice lies not in *what* exactly you do, more so *how* you are doing it.

The ability to copy what you see is not so valuable as the ability to get there on your own. To that end, we will also discuss some of the behind the scenes internal work in the Nei Gong chapter (page 93).

Neutral Stance

In the Neutral Stance we are working on letting the body relax as much as possible while still remaining upright. Through proper bone alignment, the weight of the body is naturally supported through the skeleton. This allows the muscles to relax, exerting only the minimum energy required to counteract gravity.

You may want to practice this in front of a mirror until you get a felt sense of how your joints are built to line up.

Start with your feet hip width apart. The knees should be over the feet, and slightly bent. Don't hyperextend (lock out) your knees, but don't bend them so much that they protrude past the toes either. The knees should feel strong but soft.

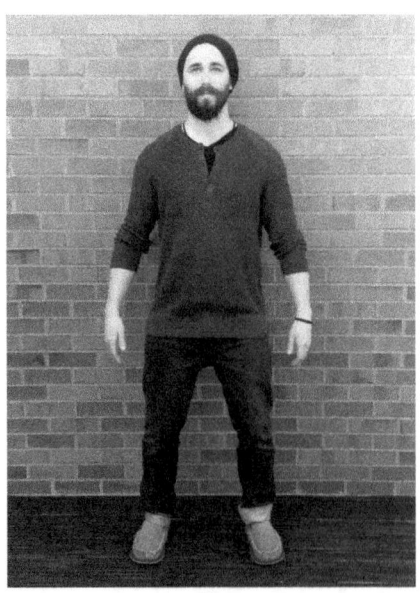

The safest place for the knees to be is directly over the toes.

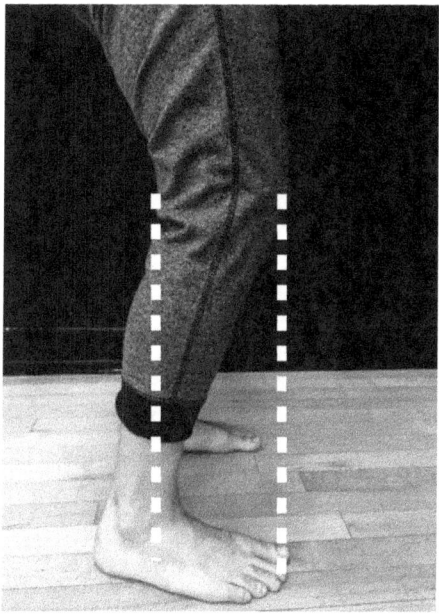

Pushing the knees too far forward will cause strain in the quads. Locking the knees backwards causes strain in the hamstrings.

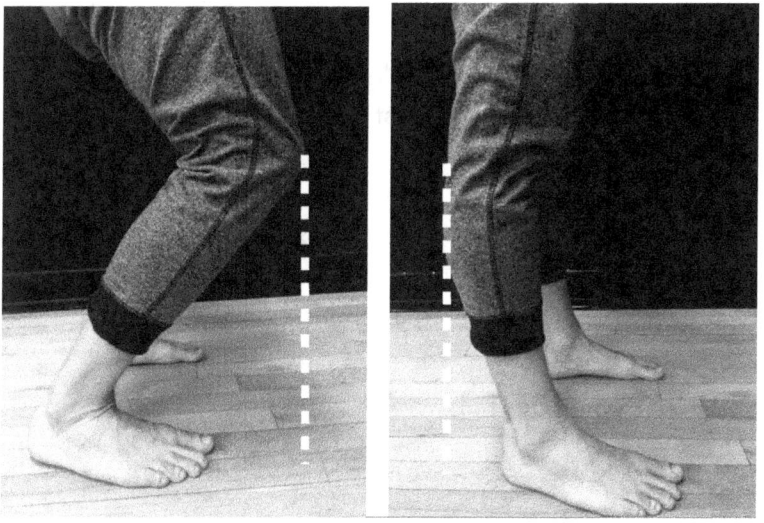

Those with flat feet will find that the knees accommodate by sinking inwards. This puts strain on the insides of the knees, and can cause pain at the medial collateral ligament, on the inside of the knee. Aligning the feet properly will help to prevent this.

Start by placing only your heel on the ground, then slowly roll the outside sole of the foot into the ground, allowing your weight to spread from the back of the foot towards the front. Slowly sink the ball of the foot into the ground, allowing the weight to spread there as well. You've just created an arch. Keeping a focus on the pinkie toe side of the ball of the foot can be helpful. Make sure that area is pressed into the ground, and it will help keep your arch from collapsing.

A common misconception of practice is that the tailbone should be tucked in. Overtucking the tailbone (like a dog tucking its tail) takes the curve out of the lower back, cramps the lower abdomen, and makes the head jut forward. This is not natural alignment. To balance the hips, it is best to think of the pelvis as a bowl of water. If you arch your lower back too much, the water will spill out of the front. If you tuck your tailbone, the water will spill out of the back. Let your hips rest naturally and evenly, so that no water would spill.

The advice to tuck your tailbone is only effective in correcting the posture when the low back gets overarched. This often happens when students are learning deep squatting postures such as Horse Stance (page 82). Even then, make sure to keep the hips level, not overtucked.

Once you have leveled your hips, imagine a weight hanging down from your tailbone, and a cord lifting up at the top of your head. In this way the spine is gently elongated, and you can express your true height. Let the muscles around your tailbone relax, and feel more of your weight pressing down through your soft knees into the earth.

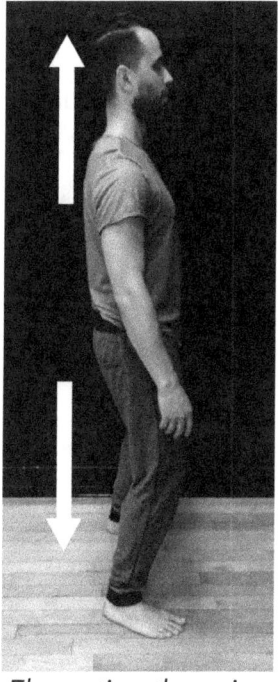

Elongating the spine.

To learn shoulder alignment, follow these four steps: Up, Back, Down, and Around. First let them scrunch up towards your ears. Then roll backwards. As you take them down the spine, the shoulders settle, but the chest puffs out. There is too much tension there. Letting the shoulders roll slightly around the sides of the body neutralizes this tension, and puts your upper body into alignment. Too much rolling will hollow out the chest, so feel your way into balance. There is a midpoint between aggressively puffing out your chest, and shrinking to protect your heart. Moving the shoulders Up, Back, Down, and Around will help you find it.

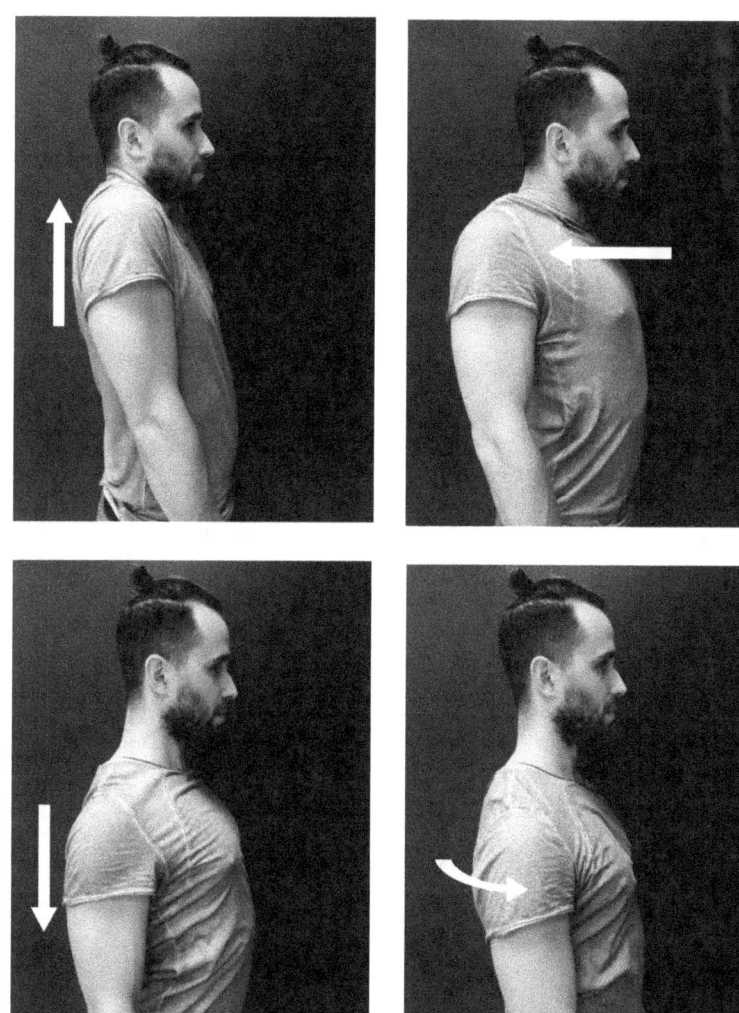

Upper Body Postures

In this section we will explore some common postures for the upper body. This is by no means an exhaustive list.

A few key points to keep in mind for the upper body:

- Keep the shoulders relaxed and down even when the arms are overhead (page 50)

- Keep a slight bend at the elbow

- Don't let the wrists kink

The postures with the hands raised overhead are generally more difficult. Similarly, postures with the palms facing inwards (Qi Ball) are much easier than palms facing outwards (Qi Bubble). Keep these points in mind when designing your practice.

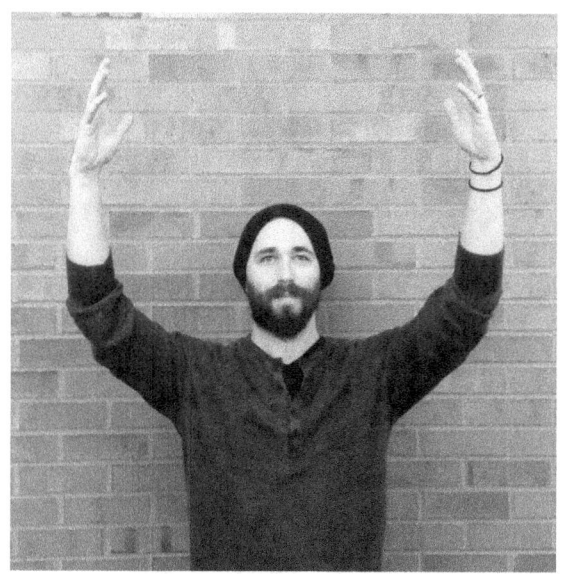

Hands high, holding the Ball.

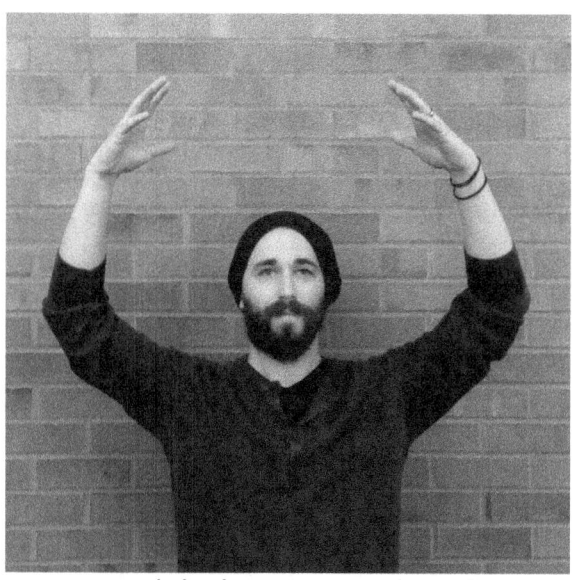

Hands high, resting on the Ball.

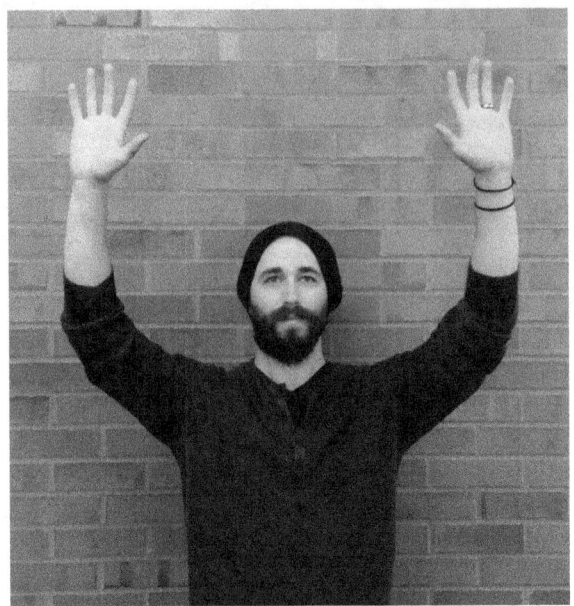

Hands high, pressing the Bubble.

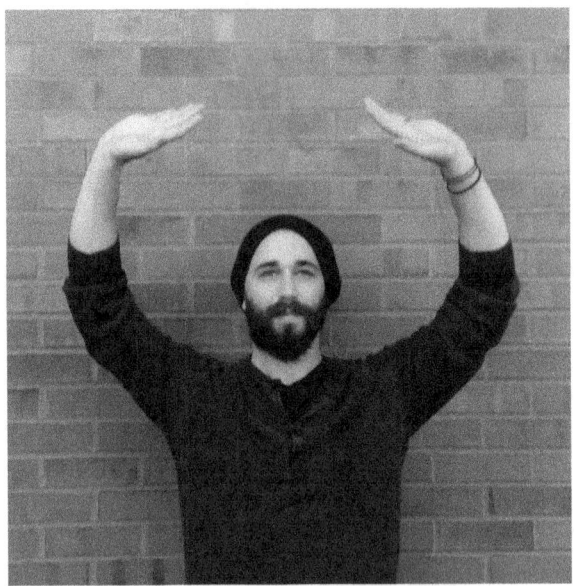

Hands high, lifting the Ball.

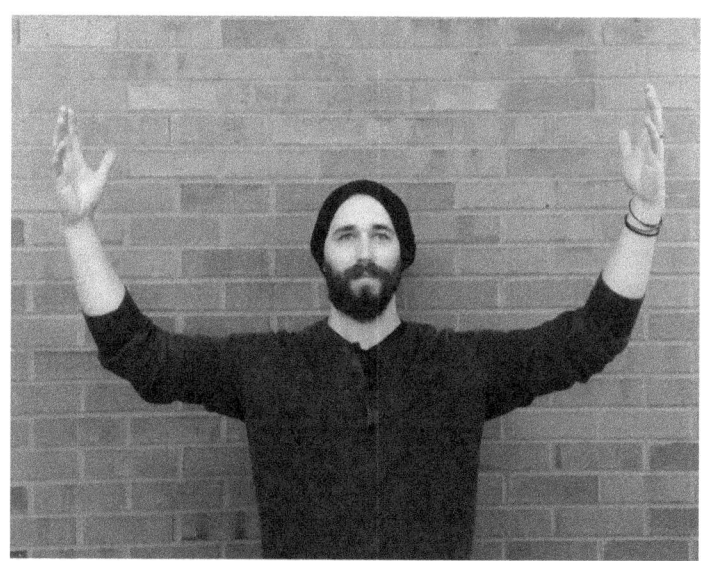

Hands high and wide, holding the Ball.

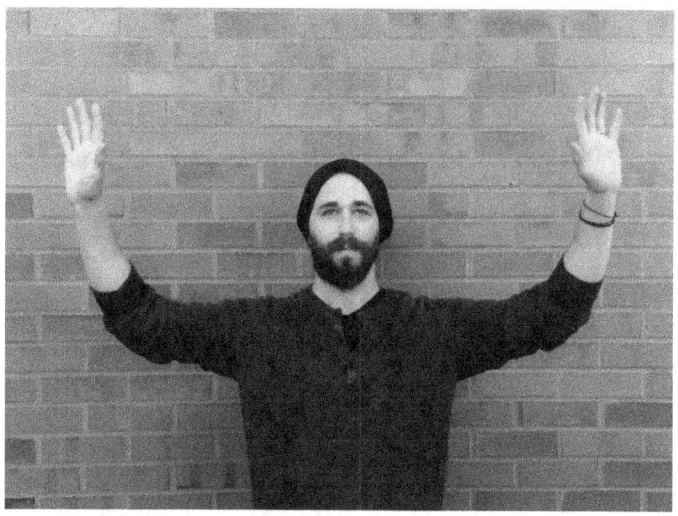

Hands high and wide, pressing the Bubble.

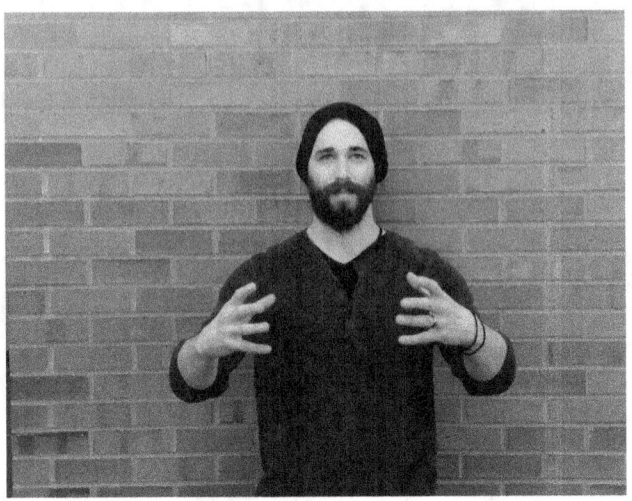

Hands chest height, holding the Ball.

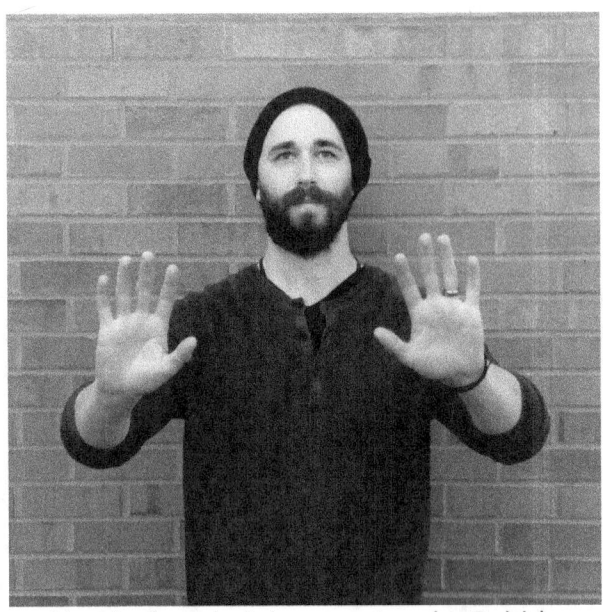

Hands chest height, pressing the Bubble.

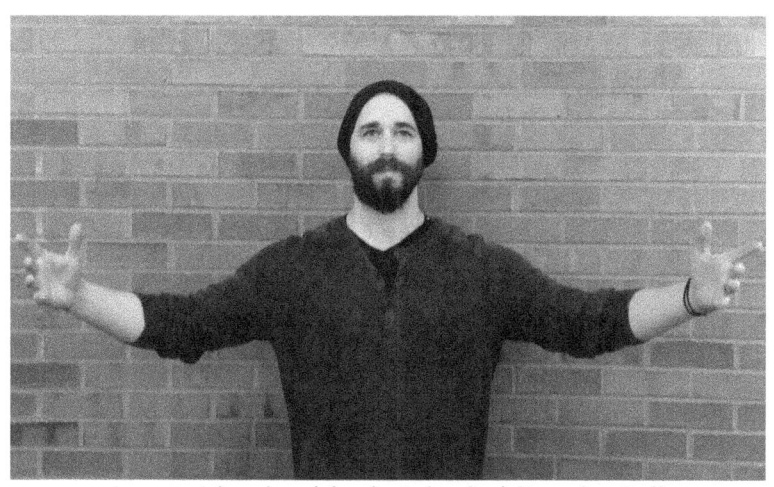

Arms wide, shoulder height, holding the Ball.

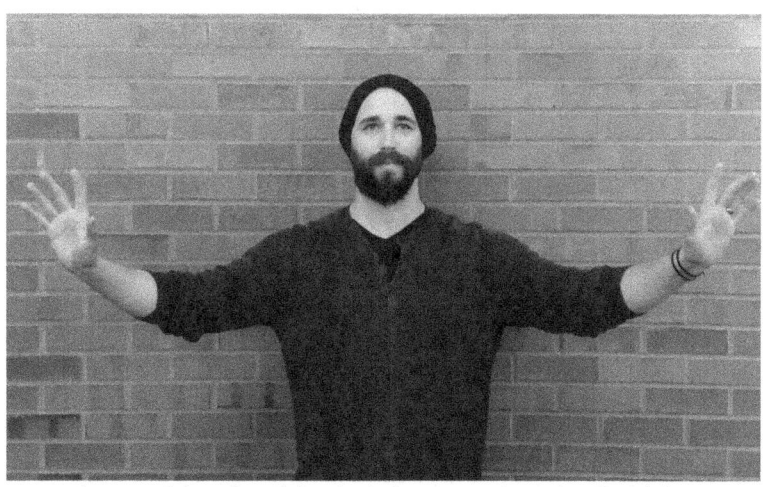

Arms wide, shoulder height, pressing the Bubble.

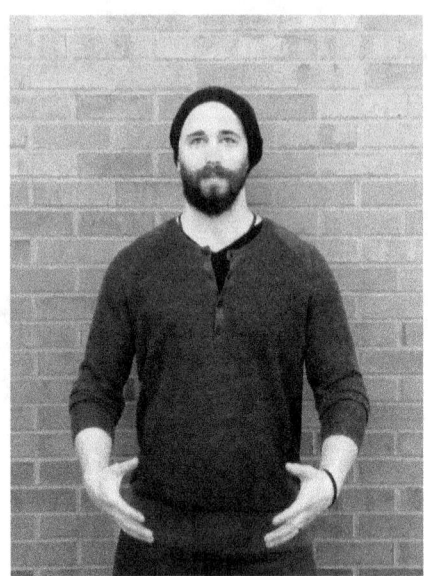

Hands at the abdomen, holding the Ball.

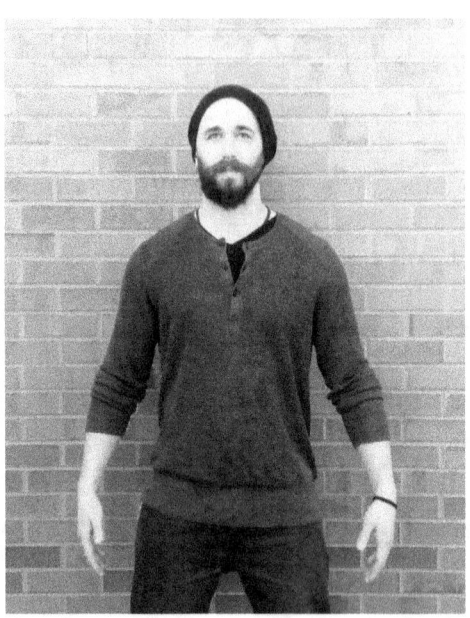

Hands at sides, palms facing inwards.

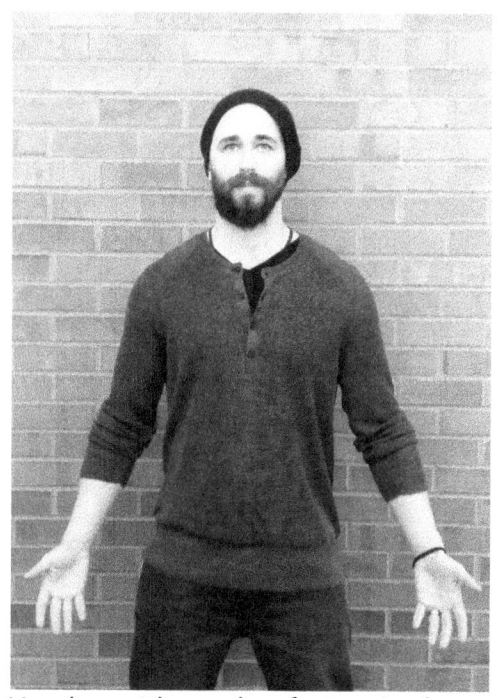

Hands at sides, palms facing the front.

Mudras

So far we've looked at open hand Qi Ball and Qi Bubble postures. Special hand shapes are called "Mudras," and there are many types. Two of my favorites are Antler Hands and the Interlocking Prayer.

Antler Hands

Keeping the hands open and expanded, bring them together so that the heels of the palms, the pads of the pinkies, and the edges of the thumbs touch.

This posture can be done with the hands at chest height, or level with the top of the head. To make it more intense, bring the forearms together as well.

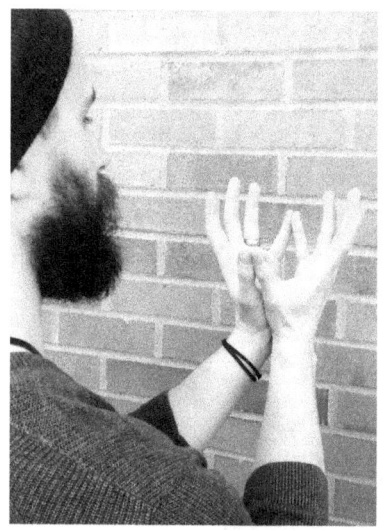 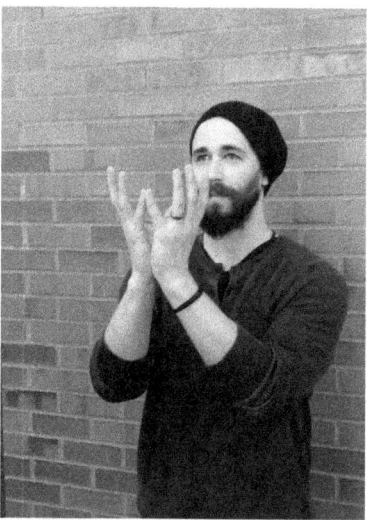

Antler Hands, two views.

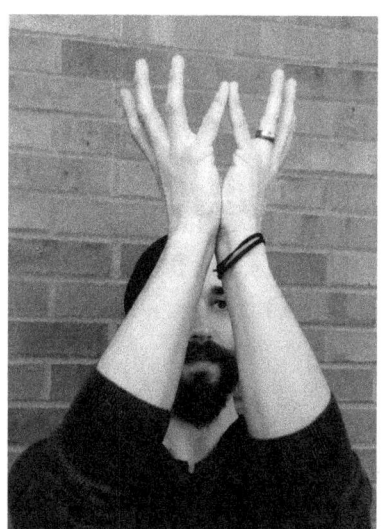 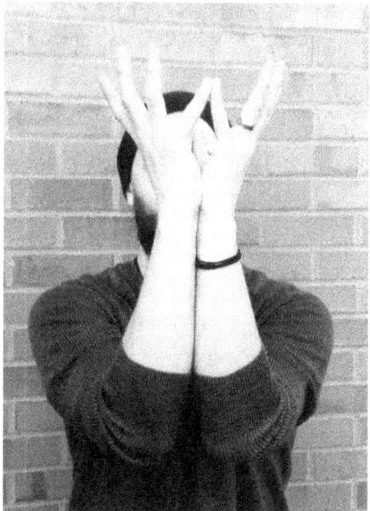

Variations: Hands overhead and forearms touching.

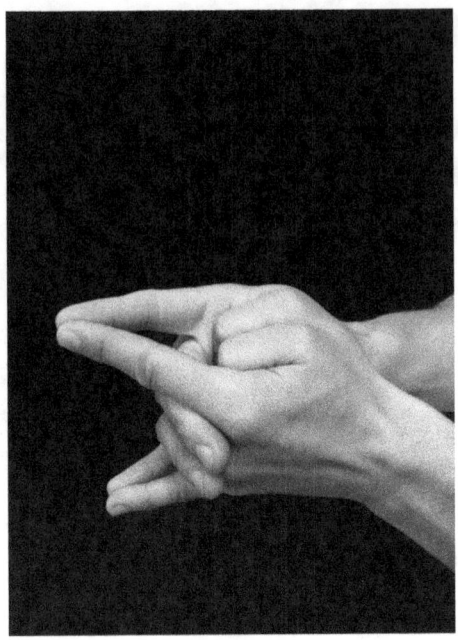

Interlocking Prayer

Begin by bringing your hands together to make an interlaced fist. Then let your pointer fingers extend and rest on each other. Next let the pinkies do the same thing. The thumbs can be crossed, or aligned along the pointer fingers with the edges touching. Tucking them inside the Mudra makes for a very solid feel as well.

We tend to have a dominant hand. When you initially interlace your fists you'll notice one side tends to go on top. Make sure you try the other arrangement as well, even though it will probably feel really odd at first.

This Mudra is especially good for overhead positions.

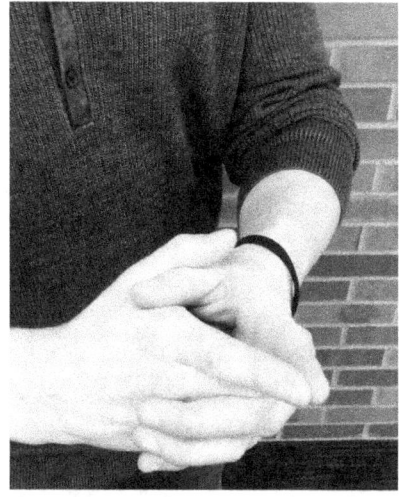
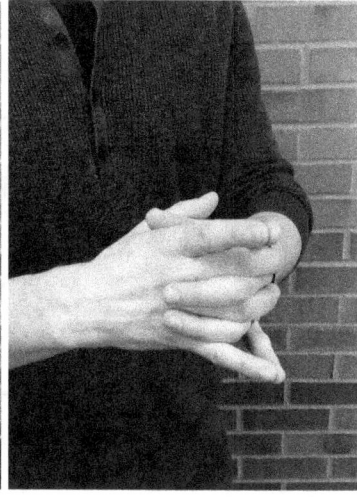
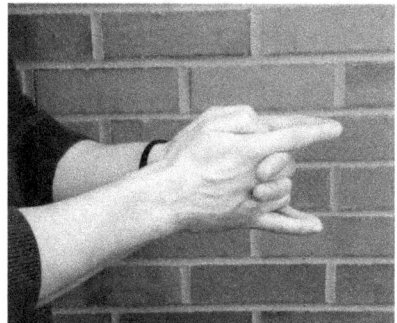

Building the Interlocking Prayer Mudra.

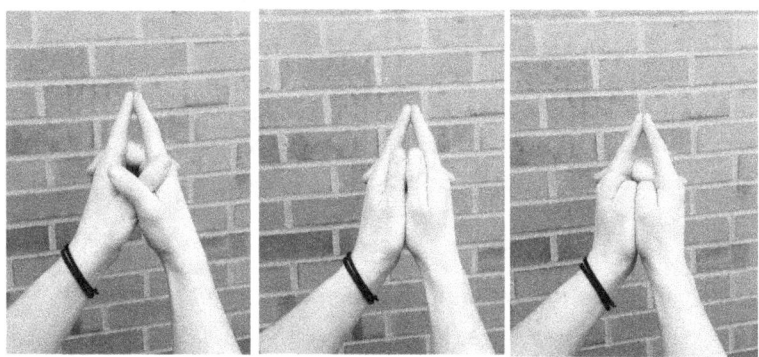

Thumbs crossed, parallel, and tucked.

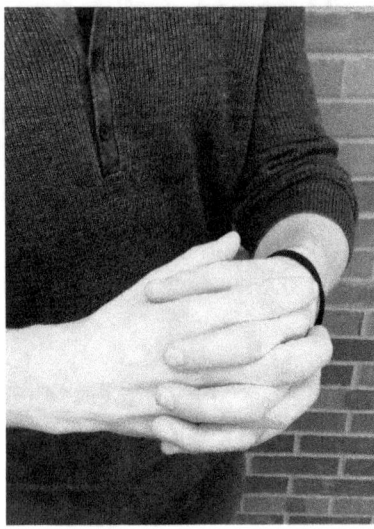
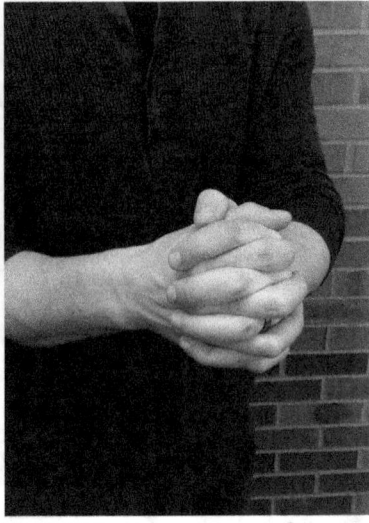

Usually the non-dominant side will feel strange at first.

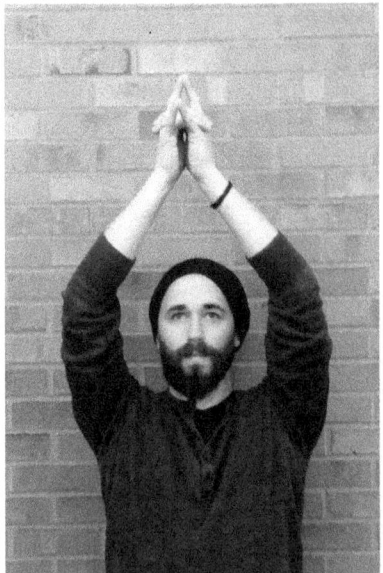
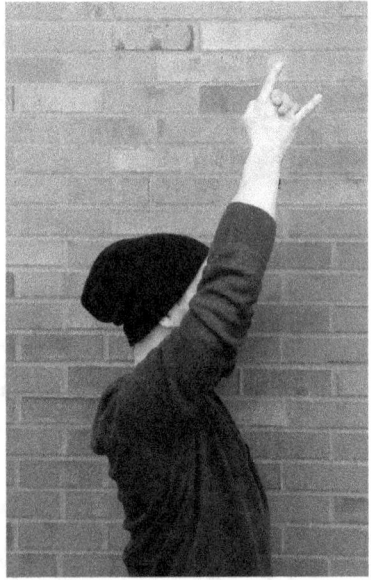

Try using the Interlocking Prayer in any overhead posture such as Tree, Warrior 1, and Warrior 3.

Lower Body Postures (Stances)

Variables that define the Stances include the distance between the feet, the angles of the feet, and weight distribution from side to side.

Things to keep in mind:

- The feet should have solid ground contact (Page 48)
- Keep the knees in line with the toes (Page 47)
- Keep the knees from locking (Page 47)
- Keep the pelvis level (Page 48)

The wider the feet are spread, the more the knees must bend, the lower the hips will drop, and the more difficult the posture. If you have knee trouble, keep the feet hip width or so until the knees get stronger.

In the Neutral Stance, the feet are hip width.

A Sinking Stance is when the feet are 1.5x hip width apart.

A Squatting Stance is when the feet are double hip width or wider.

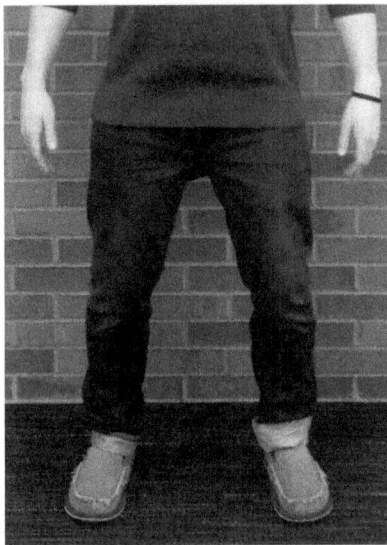
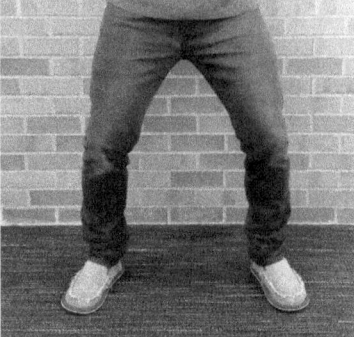
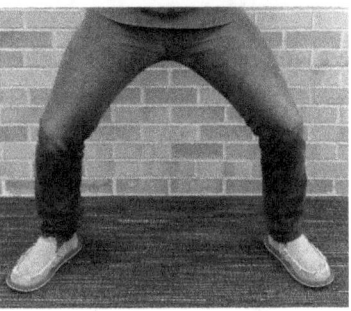

Symmetrical stances with feet hip width, 1.5x hip width, and double hip width.

Asymmetrical Lunge variations:

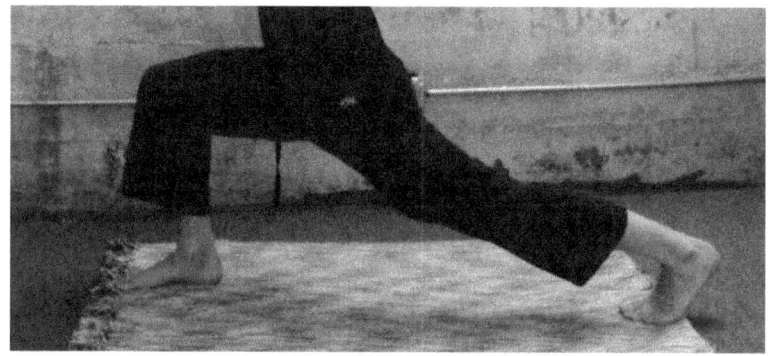

Straight Lunge (back toes facing forward).

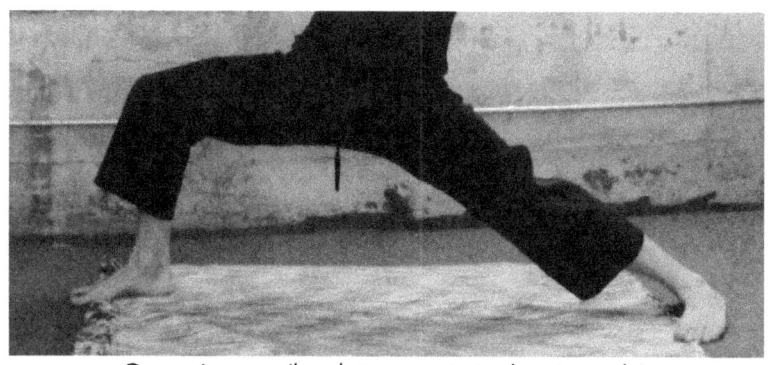

Open Lunge (back toes rotated outwards).

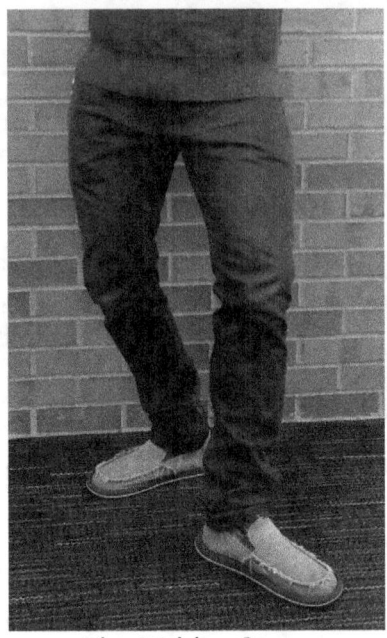

The Hidden Step:
A shallow Open Lunge with a hip-width foot distance.

A Note on Balance

Commonly, good balance is often attributed to the development of tiny "stabilization muscles." While this may be part of the story, the more the body is structurally aligned, the less muscular effort is required to counteract gravity. This type of practice develops alignment and balance over time. In order to accelerate the process, it is helpful to keep in mind a concept called "Head-Knee-Toe."

The term "Head-Knee-Toe" has to do with the vertical alignment of these three landmarks. In short, if you're standing on one foot, keep your head over that foot, with your knee between. As the knee or the head deviate from this line, it becomes much more difficult to stay upright. As usual, keep a slight bend in the knee. Try to avoid locking it, or pushing it past the toes.

Additionally, keep your centerline (your heart) pointed the same way the toes are. Having a twist in the upper body will make it more difficult to balance, especially in the more challenging positions.

Tree Pose is a classic Yoga stance that helps to train your balance. There are many variations of Tree Pose, but the common theme is that you maintain a stance on one foot.

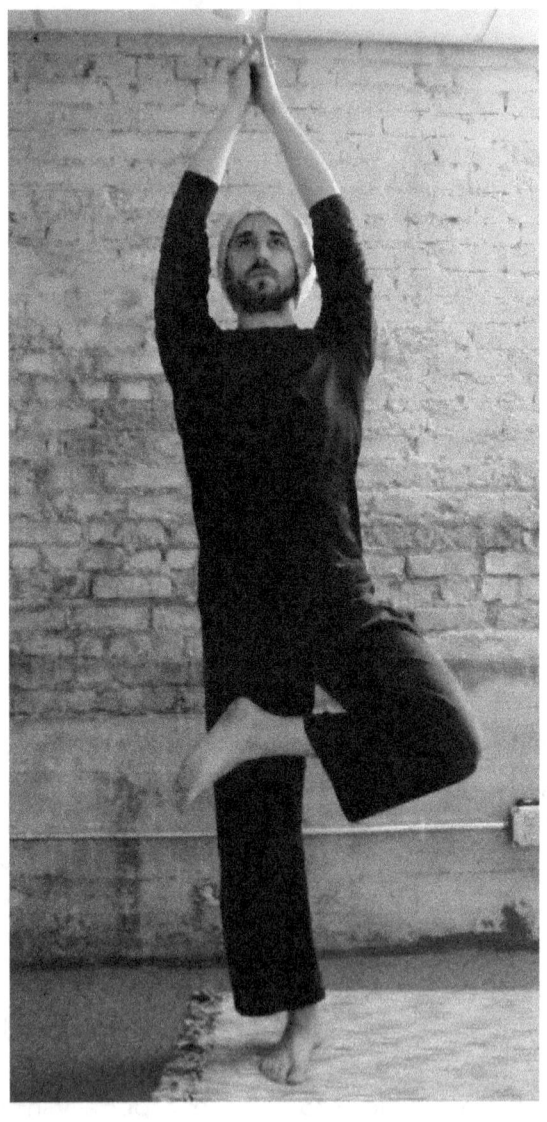

Tree Pose is much easier with a Head-Knee-Toe awareness.

Warrior 3 is another classic Yoga posture designed to develop balance. This is a posture that is also especially essential when learning Jujitsu. All beginners, and nearly all intermediate students really struggle with this posture.

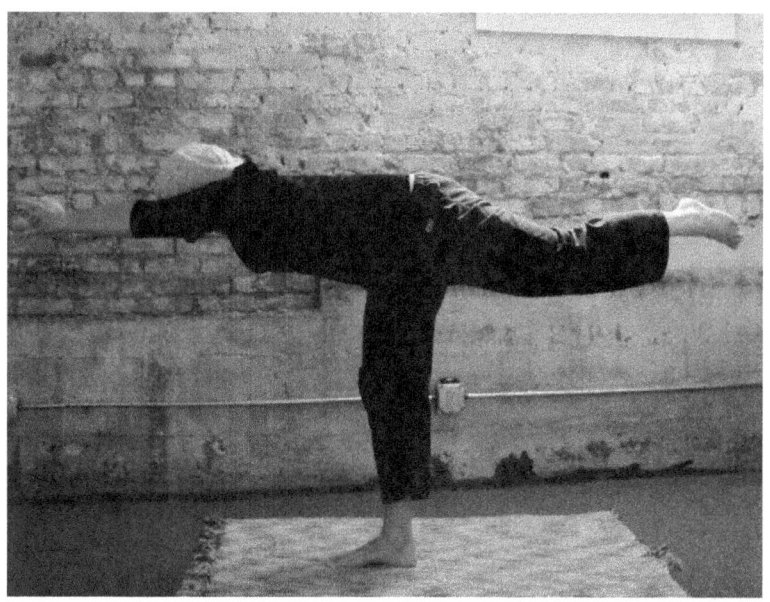

When you practice Warrior 3, make sure that you maintain the Head-Knee-Toe alignment. Also, imagine your supporting foot is on a ski, and keep your center (heart) pointed at the imaginary ski line.

These two adjustments will dramatically accelerate your progress with this posture.

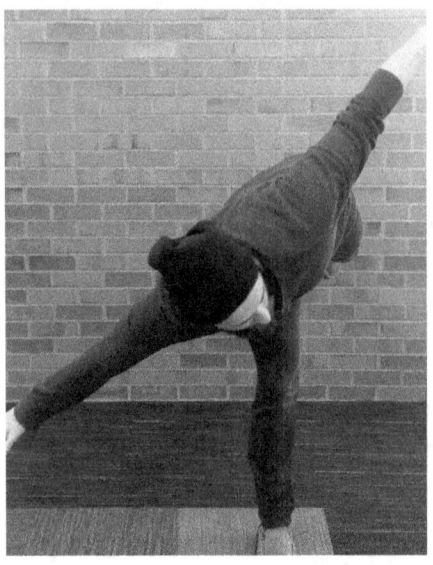

If the trunk "turns out" from the supporting leg, the midline (belt buckle, heart, nose, etc.) will point out and away from the imaginary ski. The center is unsupported.

This alignment is wobbly at best, and especially difficult to maintain. It was hard for me to hold still for the photo in this awkward position.

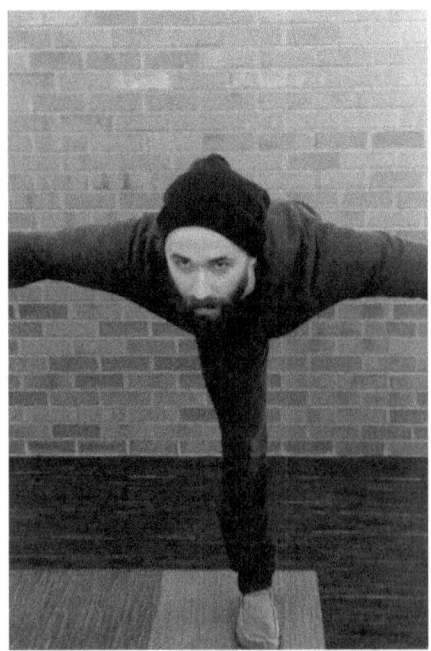

When the midline is centered over the imaginary ski, the Head-Knee-Toe alignment is emphasized. The center points downward, and the arms are even.

These adjustments are vital for balance, and will vastly improve any martial art that involves rolling, falling, or throwing.

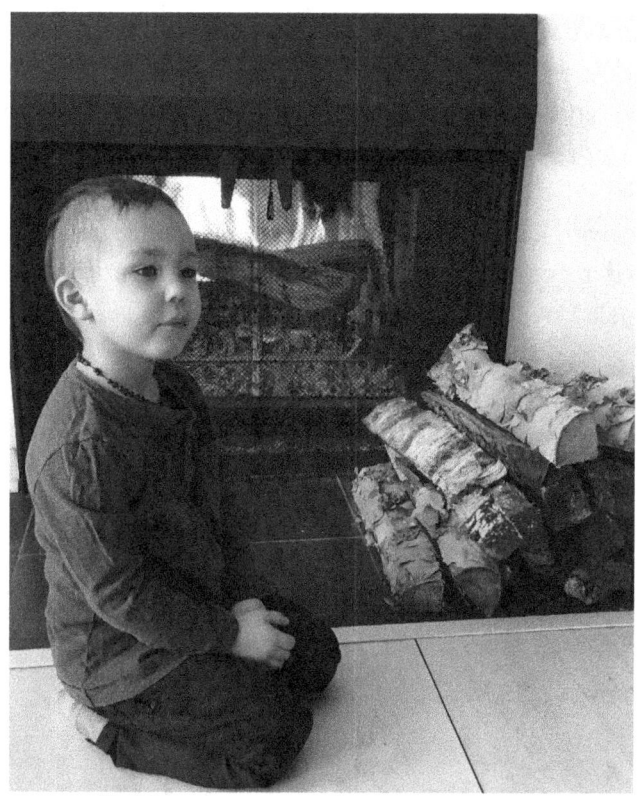

Children are naturals at sitting Seiza.

Seiza

Though not technically a stance, I feel the need to include Seiza in the list of lower body postures based on my positive experiences with it. The Japanese "Seiza" translates as "Proper Sitting."

Unless you've been doing this all your life, this posture may take some getting used to. It will become easier though with time. As usual, if you have an injury that prevents you from doing this, I highly recommend finding ways to strengthen that area (such as acupuncture, herbs, other stances) first.

In Jujitsu training we differentiate between "Live Toes" and "Dead Toes." Sitting with Live Toes makes the feet more supple, and allows you to stack the buttocks onto the heels for support. It is also a more ready position.

Sitting with Dead Toes, you may cross one big toe over the other if it's comfortable. The internal rotation of the feet creates a bowl for your hips to rest in.

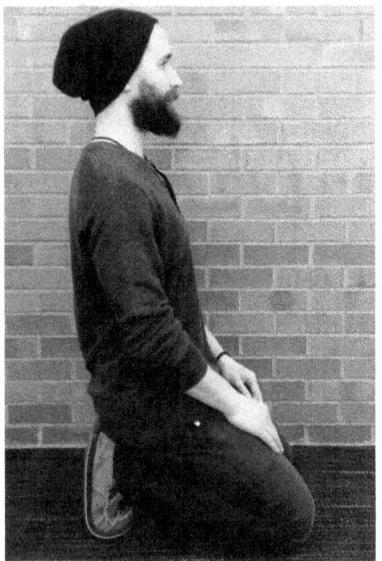 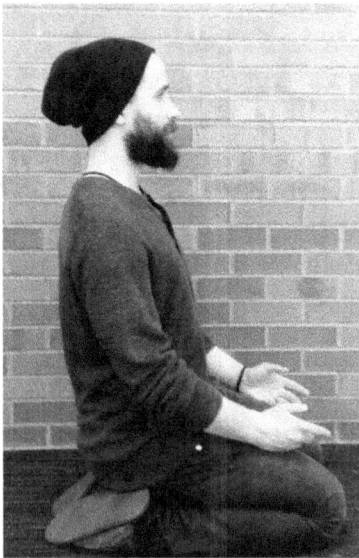

Seiza Options: "Live Toes" (Left) and "Dead Toes" (Right).

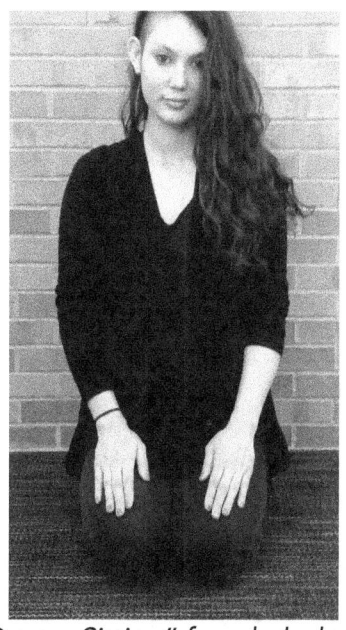

Traditional "Proper Sitting" for a lady, knees together.

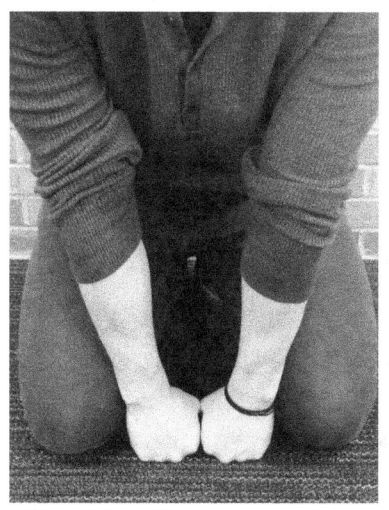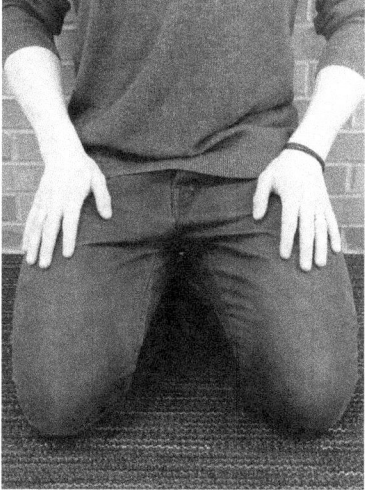

Traditionally men should leave a space of two fists' width between the knees.

Seiza is a great posture for seated meditation, breathing exercises, Qi Gong practice, etc. Try combining it with any of the upper body hand positions.

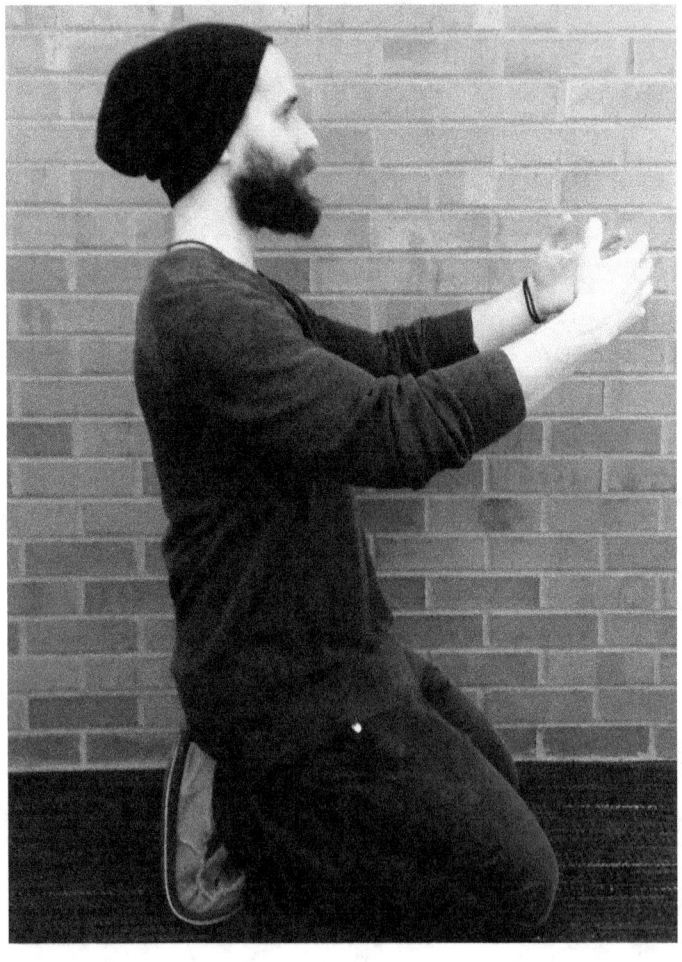

Combinations

Now that we have explored some postures for the upper and lower body, we can simply combine them to create a Standing Posture. I suggest picking your Stance first. Make sure the feet are solid. Build up from that foundation. Knees aligned. Hips level.

The connection between your legs and your arms is your spine, which rests in your hips. Maintain integrity in the core. Building up from there the shoulders should be open, head and neck aligned. Let the arms and hands bloom from the stable base of your entire body.

In general, asymmetrical postures are more advanced. A few ways to create asymmetrical postures include:

- Mixing Upper Body Postures (example: one hand overhead holding the ball, the other at abdomen height holding the ball)

- Twisting at the waist.

- Use an inherently asymmetrical Stance (Lunge, Hidden Step, Balancing).

Make sure that you split your practice time so that you can spend the same amount on each side.

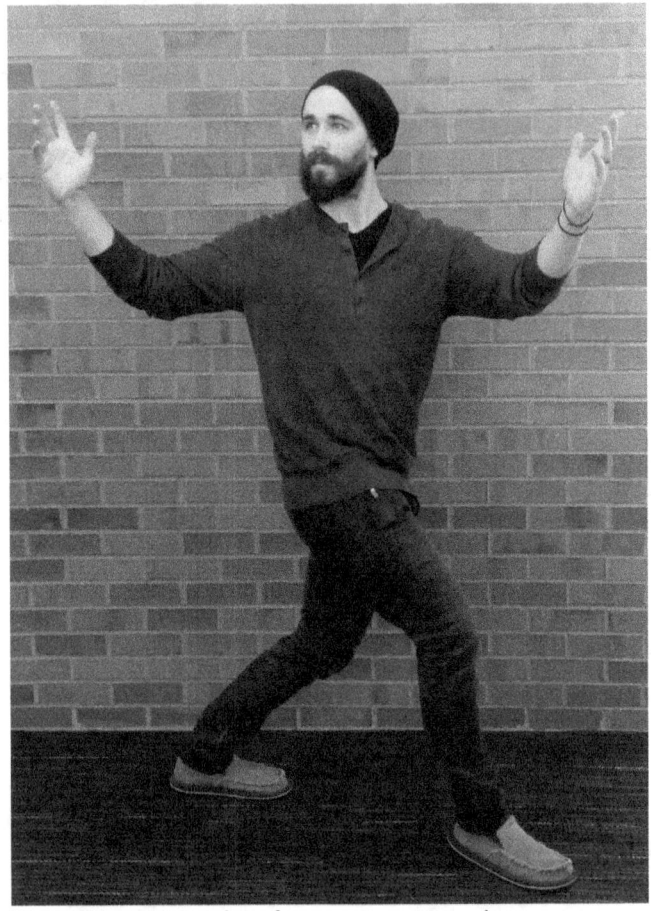

One example of an asymmetrical posture.

Special Postures

We've looked at the building blocks of the postures, and now we know how to combine them. This way we don't have to learn a million different postures in order to have a good practice.

Remember when we talked about sandwiches? Some combinations work so well that they got their own name and became famous. The Reuben, Club, BLT etc. Similarly, there are a few special postures that have really stuck with me, and I'd like to share them here with you.

Standing on Stake

This posture is one of the most fundamental. If you were to only practice one Posture in this book this would be the one.

Begin in your Neutral Stance. Feet shoulder width, knees soft, hips slightly dropped. Weight evenly split. The spine is long. The shoulders are relaxed, and the hands are about chest height, holding a Qi Ball. Elbows hang softly, and the wrists are aligned. Hands are open and relaxed.

Breathe softly from the belly.

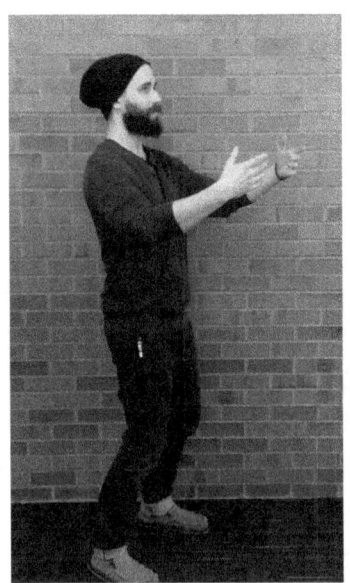 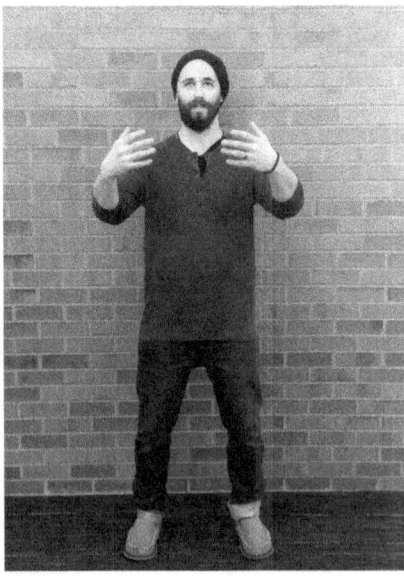

Standing on Stake, one of my top favorites.

It's important to let the arms be round. Some people like to visualize that they are hugging a tree in this position to help round out the arms. I've found that actually causes the shoulders to come forward, creating discomfort.

Instead of making the insides of the arms and chest round, try focusing the roundness on the outsides of the arms, shoulders and back. This is more like imagining being inside a hollow tree that cradles your body. It will make the practice much easier.

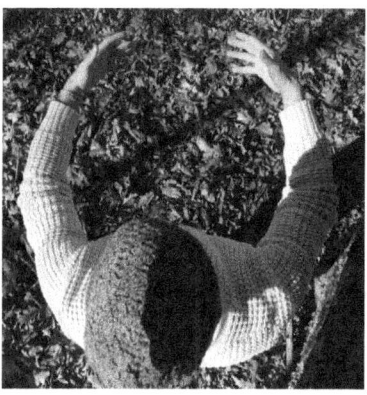

Creating roundness on the outsides of the arms and back.

Horse Stance

Horse Stance is a double shoulder width stance with the spine straight. This posture is typically considered "Hard Style," and is designed to build strength in the legs and hips.

To practice Horse Stance, step wide so that the space between your feet is double shoulder width. Let the knees bend, and the hips sink, as if you were sitting on a chair, or riding a big horse. The toes can point slightly outwards, 22.5-45°.

As the hips sink, the spine becomes long and tall, so that your chest can naturally open. Make sure that your hips drop straight down, and that your lower back doesn't overarch. Overarching causes your butt to stick out, and the back of your neck to kink. Also it creates kinks on the insides of the hips.

There are a variety of arm positions that you can use. The most advanced position requires holding the arms over the head. Intermediate position is to hold the hands out at chest height, either at the front or sides of the body. Beginners should start with the hands holding a Qi Ball at the level of the navel.

The advanced and intermediate positions can be made a little easier by letting the hands touch, as in Interlocking Prayer (page 62). The beginner position can be made easier by placing the palms on the tops of the thighs, near the knees. This takes some of the weight through the arms, and off of the upper legs.

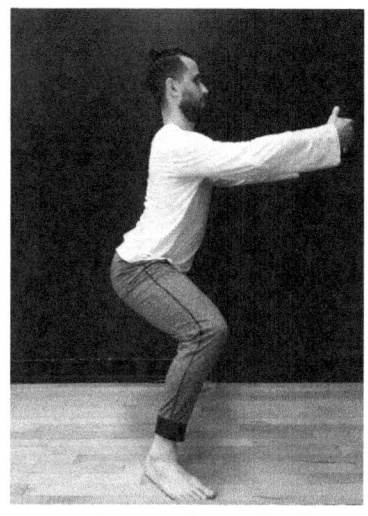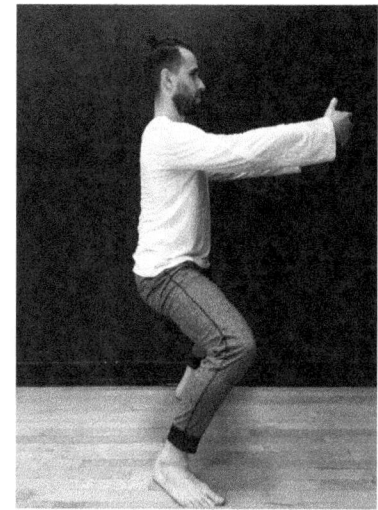

Overarching the lower back causes the dreaded "Duckbutt" (Left). Keep the pelvis level by drawing the pubic bone slightly up, and the lower ribs slightly in (Right).

A good goal is to be able to stand in Horse Stance for two minutes. You may have to work up to this, first getting comfortable with 10 seconds, 30 seconds, etc, and steadily increasing the time. Once you can do two minutes, you might aim for five or ten.

Horse Stance is by nature a challenging posture. When you feel the fire in your legs, breathe deeply and imagine sending energy there to soften them. Endurance is developed over time; use your best judgment to decide when to stand up and come out of the stance. When you do come out of your Horse Stance, keep your composure. Slowly let your arms return to your sides, and then gently stretch and shake out each leg.

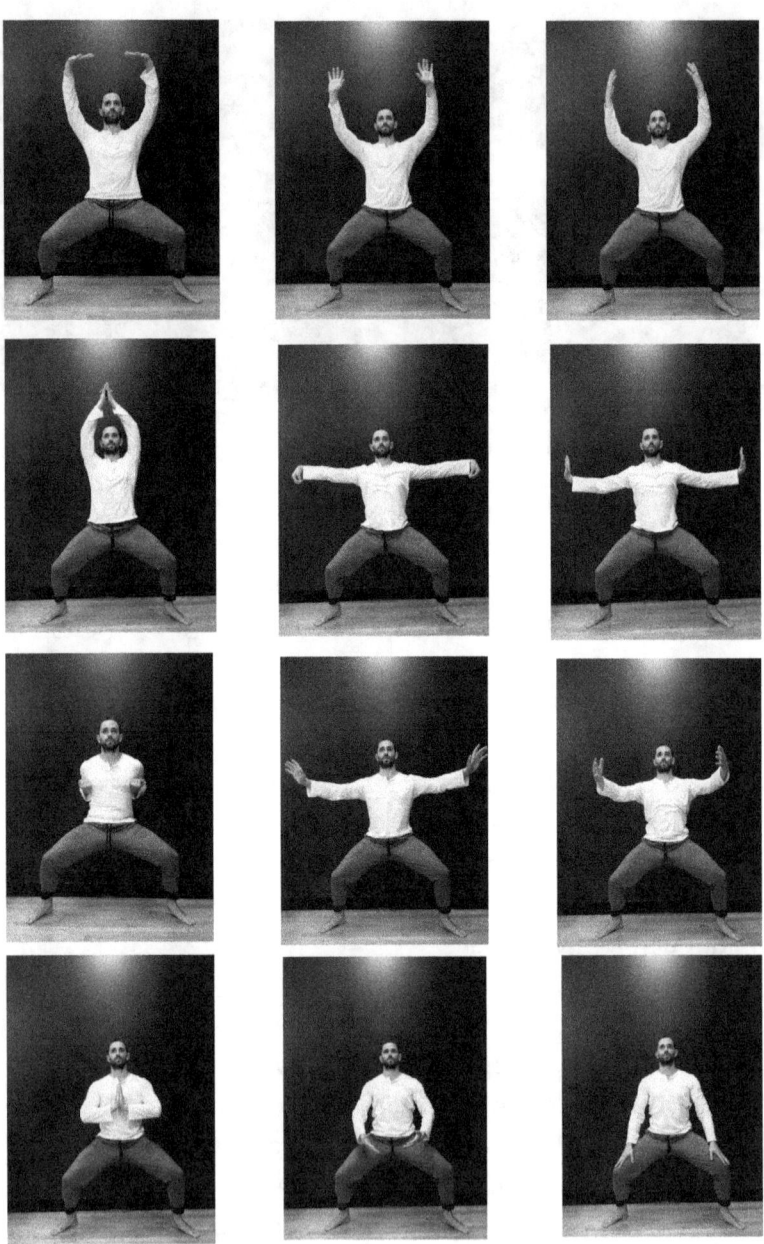

Various upper body postures to use with Horse Stance, from hardest to easiest.

If you have any pain that limits you, take it easy with this one. A great way to work into Horse Stance is to stack up a bunch of magazines, until the pile is high enough that you can sit on it, but not so high that your feet come off the floor. Every day make it a point to spend two minutes sitting on the pile of magazines. Over time, begin to remove the magazines, one at a time, until you can support yourself in the Horse Stance.

Another way to build your Horse Stance is to do it every time you brush your teeth. Bring the training home and integrate it into your life for best results.

Practicing Horse Stance in this way will build up strength in the knees and legs, as well as in the lower back. It can also help to soothe anxiety or a racing mind.

Some schools practice their Horse Stance extremely low, with the hips at the same height or even lower than the knees. In this way the thighs are level with the ground, and a staff can be balanced there without rolling off. An old Kung Fu teacher of mine used to train the class in this way. He would also walk around the room swinging a long staff around to make sure your head was low enough. If anyone's stick rolled off of their legs, the whole class had to start the exercise over. That's one way to train, old school.

Dropping the hips that low challenges the legs a lot more. Unfortunately, it also tends to make it difficult to keep the spine upright without overarching the back, and kinking the hips and neck. If you would like to get the benefit of the low stance, without sacrificing your frame, try the Tortoise (page 87).

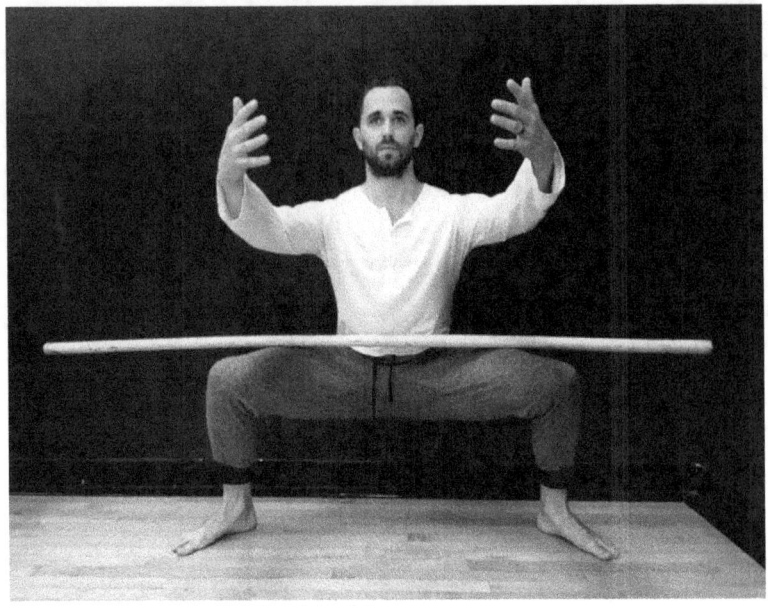

Old school horse stance.

Tortoise

The Tortoise is a variation of Horse Stance. To practice the Tortoise, begin with feet double shoulder width. The feet may turn outwards 22.5-45°. As you let your knees bend, sink your hips deeply, until they are level with, or slightly below the knees. Keeping your spine elongated, fold your torso forward so that your chest is pointing to the ground. Keep your neck aligned, and let your eyes gaze softly at the ground. Bring your hands together at your chest with the palms, edges, or backsides of the hands touching.

Breathe smoothly in this position, and work up to holding it for a few minutes. Remember to let your hips sink, stretch and relax.

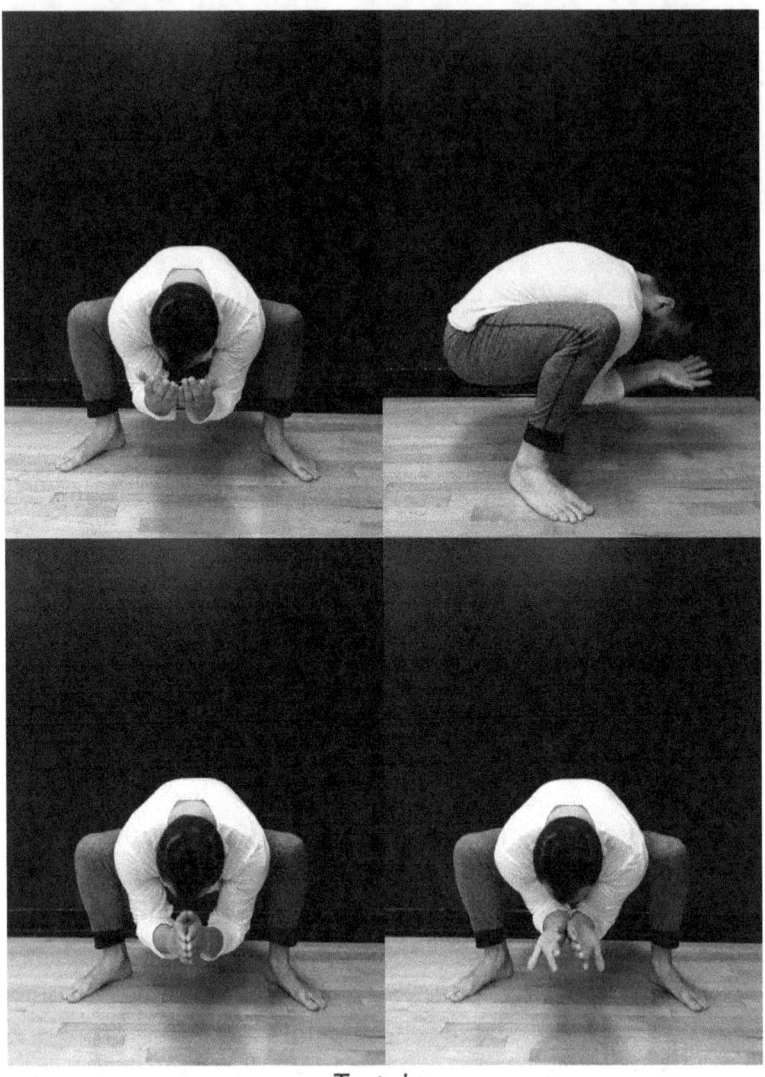

Tortoise.

Bird of Prey

The Bird of Prey is an advanced posture that helps with balance and flexibility. Begin in your neutral stance, and slowly shift all of your weight onto your right foot. As the left foot becomes free, lift it up, and set the outside of the left ankle on the right thigh, just above the knee.

Once the left foot is in place, bend the right knee, and sink the hips. Don't let the low back overarch, though the spine will lean forward a bit in this posture. Look straight ahead, and send both the arms out to the sides and behind the back, letting all five fingertips come together, or whatever else you'd like to do with your hands.

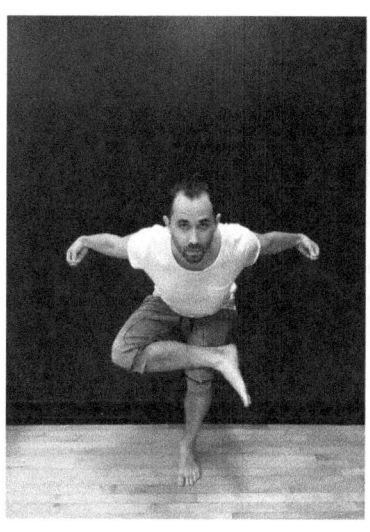
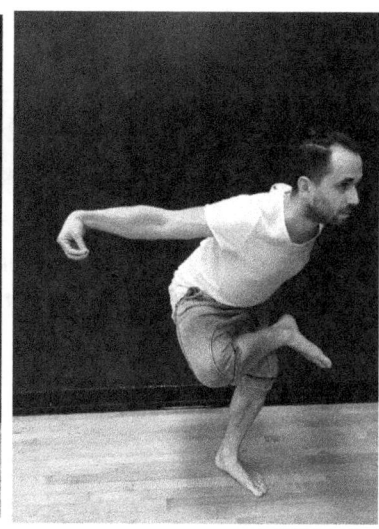

Hold this position for at least six deep breaths. Try to work your way up to two minutes. Then repeat on the other side.

If you don't have enough balance or flexibility to get into this position, there are two Yoga postures that will help prepare you: Tree (page 70) and Pigeon (Below).

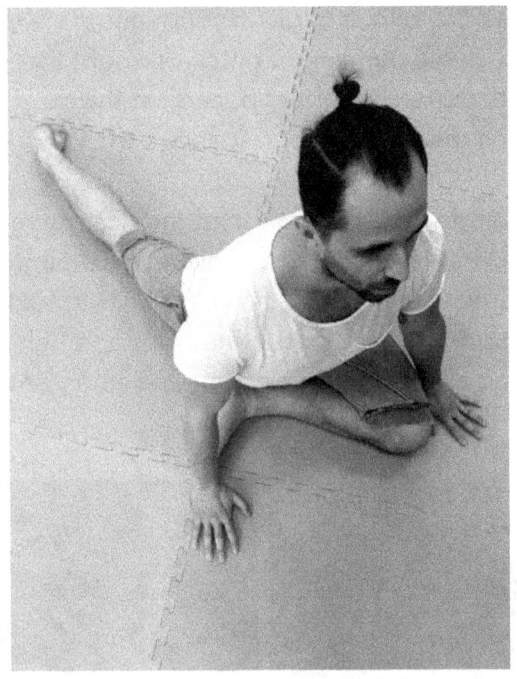

Good prep for the hip flexibility required for Bird of Prey. Flexible hips help keep the low back pain free.

Saito Dragon

This is an exercise that stretches and strengthens the lower body, while expanding and opening the upper body. To practice, start in a deep Straight Lunge. As you sink your hips into the lunge, let your spine elongate, and become internally expanded. Open your arms out to the sides as far as possible without kinking the shoulders, fingers open, palms facing forwards, pressing a gigantic Qi Ball. Let your eyes open as much as possible, and direct your gaze forwards.

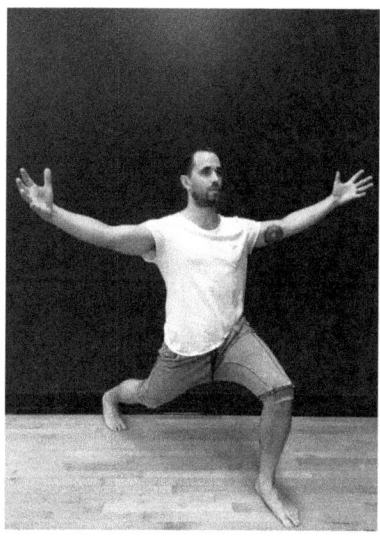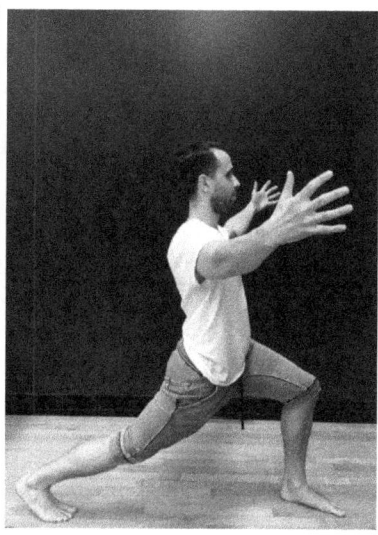

While in this position, allow your lower body to stabilize and root to the center of the Earth. Your upper body expands and radiates. Imagine energy coming out of your heart and eyes, filling the space around you. Own the space. Maintain that intensity while you breathe smoothly and deeply. Hold this posture, then repeat on the other side. Work up to being able to practice this for five minutes on each side. Consider it a test of willpower.

Nei Gong

Nei Gong

So far we've explored the mechanics of the Standing Postures. The physical form is only the foundation for practice. When we add elements of visualization, micromovements, and internal awareness, this practice really takes on a life of its own.

There are four steps of Nei Gong ("internal practice"):

Opening
Keeping the posture aligned, not kinked. Keeping the blood flow smooth. Warming Up. Stretching. Eating well.

Connecting
Learning to access energy from very big sources (the center of the Earth for example).

Gathering
Learning methods to draw the energy from the big source into the body.

Directing
Sending the accumulated energy somewhere for a specific purpose.

Rooting

Rooting is the process of expanding your energetic awareness beyond the boundaries of your feet and into the Earth. From a grounded stance, pay attention to the way the Earth feels as it presses back up into your feet. Imagine the boundary between your body and the Earth slowly dissolving, until you can feel some of your awareness penetrate the Earth.

Extend that awareness deeper and deeper into the ground. Sometimes it helps to imagine energetic roots coming out of your feet, digging their way through the Earth. You might start out a few inches deep, then a few feet. Maybe you can feel into the Earth a distance equivalent to your height. From there, gradually deepen that sense to two body heights, ten body heights, etc. Ultimately, imagine that your energetic roots extend extremely deep, all the way to the center of the Earth.

You might imagine the center of the Earth as a swirling mass of near infinite light and energy. Connecting to this power source through Rooting will dramatically enhance the effects of your practice.

Waving the Spine

As you inhale, let the weight shift forward to the balls of the feet. Notice how the knees naturally want to move slightly forward. As the knees advance, the hips press forward, and the pelvis rolls forwards, slightly arching the lower back. The arch of the lower back sends a wave up through each vertebra that causes the chest to open. The opening of the chest naturally rolls the shoulders down, which effortlessly allows the elbows and hands to float slightly upwards.

This process is reversed during the exhalation. The weight rolls back to the heels, the knees shift back slightly (staying bent, not locked), the pelvis rolls backwards allowing the sacrum to tuck slightly, taking the arch out of the lower back. Next the upper back rounds ever so slightly, and the hands naturally glide toward the floor.

The waving motion causes the spine to extend slightly during the inhalation, and flex slightly during the exhalation. You'll know you're on the right track when the wave motion connects from the feet all the way to the head and the hands, and slight raising and lowering happen on their own as you relax into the gentle wave.

As you become comfortable with this movement, start reducing the amplitude of the wave. Making your movements smaller and smaller, until they are almost imperceptible will enhance the internal sensations greatly.

Standing perfectly still is difficult. Connecting to an imperceptible waving motion that follows the breath brings this practice to life. These types of Micromovements are what makes this type of practice so attainable and vivid.

Be persistent while learning to Wave the Spine. It may take a while to feel connected and comfortable, but learning to smoothly integrate your entire body, first with the big wave, and then the small wave, is extremely rewarding.

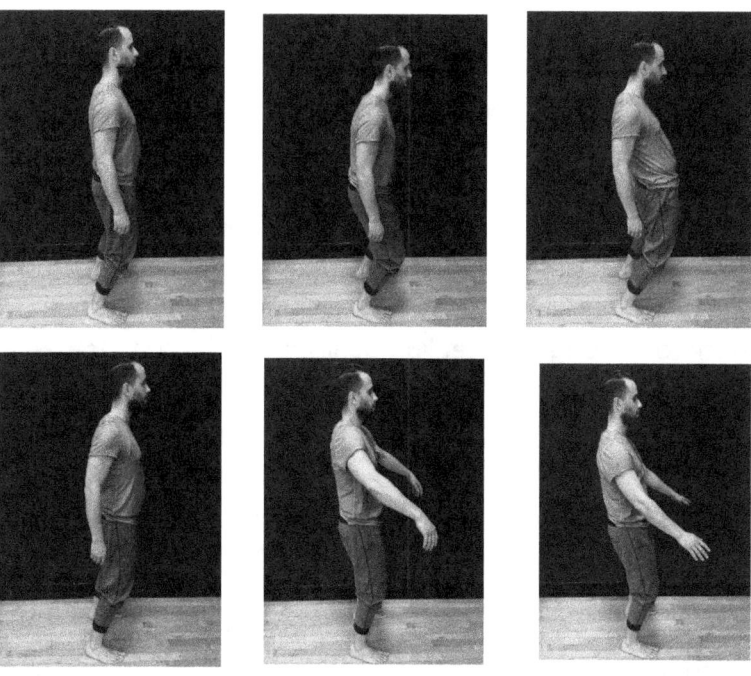

Micromovements

It's easiest to learn movements when they are very large and exaggerated. As you get the feel for any motion, try making the movements smaller and slower. To an outside observer, it would be difficult to detect the motion; you almost appear still. Internally, however, the effects are profound. Less is more, as you'll discover by making your movements smaller and slower.

Try holding the Qi Ball while standing. As before, you can match the rhythm of the breath to the expansion and compression of the ball. Begin by inhaling and expanding the ball a few inches on either side. Exhale and press it back to the original size. Gradually make the distance smaller, so you expand the ball by one inch during the inhalation, and then press it back to its original size on the exhalation. See what the smallest distance you can cover is. Can you move only one centimeter over the course of a breath cycle? One millimeter? To cover less distance, the physical movements must become much slower. Notice how the less you move the more intense the energy becomes.

As a contrast, try to stand still, and not move the hands at all. Most people find Micromovements to be dramatically easier than standing still, and much more profound in terms of Qi generation.

Try sending your roots to the center of the Earth; as you inhale, imagine energy coming up through your roots, through your feet, subtly waving through your spine, and filling the ball as it gently expands. The exhalation is a chance for the hands to lightly press into the surface of the energy ball, as the spine settles back to slight flexion, and the energy distributes itself within and around your body.

Directing

As you learn to connect to the ground, and gather energy up into your body through your feet, the next step is to direct it. Very simply, use your mind to guide the energy through your entire body, filling every cell with white light.

Once you feel full, continue drawing energy up from the ground, guide it through your body, and direct it to your palms. If you are holding a Qi Ball, fill the space with that energy. If you are pressing into a Qi Bubble, send the energy to the surface of the Bubble.

Directing has many applications- healing, striking, manifestation, even simple tasks like shaking coffee grounds out of a french press. Successful Directing is the end result of the other foundational Nei Gong practices of Opening, Connecting, and Gathering.

Mist on the Mountain

Mist on the Mountain is an image to help keep the foundation sturdy and the arms soft.

While standing, imagine your lower body is sitting on a mountaintop. Your legs provide a relaxed stability. Consciously relax the muscles around your tailbone and feel your feet press into the ground more solidly.

Use Rooting to connect down into the center of the Earth, and a Micromovement version of Waving the Spine to subtly draw the energy up during the inhalations. Feel your spine flex and extend a millimeter at a time during the respiratory cycle. Notice how your arms expand and compress one millimeter at a time. This motion follows your breath, which is smooth and soft.

As your lower body sits on the mountain, imagine your upper body is a mist. Let your arms be as soft and loose as possible. As you exhale, direct the energy into the palms and outward from there.

Shen Gong

Shen Gong

Standing practice is a contemplation on stillness. By slowing down the body and the breath, the mind will follow. "Shen Gong" translates as "Spiritual Cultivation." I use this term to describe the mental side of this type of training.

It is helpful here to understand some of the different aspects of our consciousness:

The **Subconscious** is the hidden aspect of our conscious that typically runs behind the scenes.

The **Narrator** is the aspect of our consciousness that is constantly telling us the story of what is going on.

The **Observer** is the aspect of our consciousness that simply listens.

The **Muse** is the voice of inspiration that may originate from the Subconscious. In the old days the Muse was thought to be an external force that visited us.

Of course this is a gross oversimplification of the mind, and these aspects are not so easy to separate. This model is very useful though in explaining some of the different phases of meditation.

Inspiration
Many people (artists, writers, entrepreneurs) use Standing practice as a way to quiet the mind in order to welcome the Muse and overcome creative blocks. The Muse usually feels unwelcome in the unrelenting chatter and judgment of the Narrator. If you stand long enough (usually 15 minutes), the Narrator begins to quiet down. At that point the environment of the mind becomes calm and pleasant. Time is of no concern. In that receptive state, we tend to find inspiration. When we get quiet, we get ideas.

Interrogation
Another level of practice, and one that can be extremely challenging, is to go beyond the Muse. Wait long enough and the voice of inspiration will quiet down too. Then you can access deeper layers of your self.

One of my favorite ways to encourage this process involves continuously asking yourself one question: *Who am I?*

Don't do this out loud. Have the dialogue in your head. As soon as the question is posed, the Narrator will rush to answer. No matter what the answer, reject it and ask again.

Keep going until the Narrator is not so quick, and you (the Observer) will start to notice the space between the question and the answer, where there is no voice.

In that space lies your answer.

Koans

Zen practitioners routinely employ the use of Koans, which are a type of riddle. Students are given illogical questions to ponder such as "What is the sound of one hand clapping?"

At first this seems like a test of cleverness. Everyone wants to find the right answer. However the actual benefit of these riddles comes not in the solution, but in the process of grinding out the question.

Consider the previous meditation, where we ask a simple question (Who am I?) and reject every answer until we get a peek at the empty stage of our minds. Koans are beautifully employed because there is no answer.

We ask impossible questions of our minds, in hopes that the space before the next answer will be as long as possible.

In that space we know ourselves.

You can do this while standing. Maybe better to sit.

Appendices

Appendix 1: Sample Sessions

This information has been presented in a way to encourage
modular thinking and customization of the practice. You
are encouraged to build your own custom Standing
Postures, and design your own sessions. What follows are
merely examples if you need help getting started.

Beginner Form
Approximately 18 minutes

Counterswing (2 minutes)
Bouncing (2 minutes)
Stretch out a bit
Horse Stance (30 seconds)
Custom: any Upper Body Posture + any Stance (3 minutes)
Standing on Stake (5 minutes)
Neutral Stance (1 minute)
Scoop the Moon (3 times)

Intermediate Form
Approximately 35 minutes

All Warmups (5 minutes)
All Dao Yin Stretches (5 Minutes)
Warrior Three (2 minutes each side)
Custom Asymmetrical Posture (2 minutes each side)
Standing on Stake (15 minutes)
Scoop the Moon (9 times)

Advanced Form
Approximately 35 minutes

All Warmups (5 minutes)
All Dao Yin Stretches (5 Minutes)
Horse Stance (3 minutes)
Standing on Stake (20 minutes)
Scoop the Moon (9 times)

Quick and Dirty Form
10-20 minutes

Standing on Stake (10-20 minutes)
Scoop the Moon (1 time)

Appendix 2: Exercise Index